SHAHROO IZADI

the
last
diet.

Discover the secret to
losing weight
FOR GOOD

bluebird
books for life

For my mum, who's proof that kindness
and strength go hand in hand.

First published 2019 by Bluebird

This paperback edition first published 2020 by Bluebird
an imprint of Pan Macmillan
The Smithson, 6 Briset Street, London EC1M 5NR
Associated companies throughout the world
www.panmacmillan.com

ISBN 978-1-5098-8338-7

1 3 5 7 9 8 6 4 2

A CIP catalogue record for this book is available from the British Library.

Typeset in Baskerville MT Std and Averta Std by
Palimpsest Book Production Ltd, Falkirk, Stirlingshire

Printed and bound by CPI Group (UK) Ltd, Croydon, CRO 4YY

Visit **www.panmacmillan.com** to read more about all our books
and to buy them. You will also find features, author interviews and
news of any author events, and you can sign up for e-newsletters
so that you're always first to hear about our new releases.

Contents

Foreword

All I wanted was for this book to convince people that they didn't need to punish themselves in order to change their eating habits and manage their weight on their own terms. I got what I wanted. And yet, the lengthy and heartfelt 'thank yous' I receive from readers are often bittersweet.

I was far too busy worrying about whether *The Last Diet* would be genuinely helpful or well received to consider that behind every message of gratitude and feedback, there would be a painful story.

A story of a young person who learned to dislike themselves and grew into an adult who had become accustomed to punishing their body. A story of someone who spent a lifetime ashamed of how they look, ashamed of their inability to manage their own habits, ashamed of the lengths they'd gone to try and change their bodies and ashamed that they didn't feel capable – or worthy – of taking the same common sense advice they'd give their loved ones.

I could never have imagined the extent to which my own story would be told back to me, and how needlessly alone I would realise I had been this whole time.

Of course I wanted readers to relate to the case studies in the book, and to find the exercises useful, but I could never have guessed how many people would relate to the most personal parts of it – and how many would tell me that they could relate to every single word.

Not only did people not judge or ridicule my experience (as I'd spent so many sleepless nights fearing), but the compassion that readers of *The Last Diet* have shown me has surpassed anything I could have hoped for or imagined in my wildest dreams. Many shared that the similarities they saw in my story helped them to find compassion for themselves. I can absolutely relate to this every time I'm overwhelmed with empathy and compassion for readers and their very familiar experiences.

Turns out, it wasn't just me who had grown accustomed to spending all day thinking about what I would (or wouldn't) eat, or replaying a constant internal soundtrack about myself and my body that was unkind and unfair. Readers now regularly share with me that they too got to a stage where they'd have chosen to change their eating habits even if the by-product wasn't weight loss, just so they could reclaim their 'brain space'.

I now know for sure that I was far from alone in feeling completely misunderstood when I'd hear people trivialise the very thing I found most challenging, but stayed quiet; assuming it was just me who had something wrong with them. Naturally, I knew that people struggled with their weight and their eating habits, of course I did. I guess deep down though, I still always assumed that the way I thought and behaved was more shameful than anyone else.

Thanks to the honest discussions that this book has facilitated, I've been able to really clarify for myself how I can be body positive and want to manage a weight that feels right for my body simultaneously. I'm now able to share some of the lengths I went to in order to be in any other body; extreme measures that I wasn't ready to talk about when this book was first published out of fear and shame.

I thought that writing *The Last Diet* would mark the end of a process for me, but the stories it's opened my eyes to have made me realise that it was in fact the beginning of a very new chapter. One where I'd find that the next step after showing myself the same compassion I show others was to learn that none of us deserve to feel shame, either. And one where I'm committed to doing whatever I can, however scary it may be, to make it so that the experiences I share in this book are one day no longer relatable.

Readers of *The Last Diet* have helped me to understand who I'm best placed to help, support and truly connect with: it's those who believe that diets not only made them like themselves less, but resulted in them gaining weight over time and not trusting themselves around food. Those who, like me, are anti diet culture and would never recommend diets to their children; who are all for intuitive eating styles and moderation, but who know that a lot of unlearning needs to happen before they can make those shifts from an authentic and honest place. Those who are caught between a world that wouldn't accept them the way they were, and is now asking them to love themselves – with urgency. Those who believe wholeheartedly that their unwanted weight comes as a direct result of being unkind to themselves and eating in ways that don't make them feel good. Those who want to learn to love food and themselves. The fact that people from all over the world now share with me that *The Last Diet* has enabled them to do just that, makes it hands down the most important thing I've created in my life.

If you're reading this and you suspect that your story might be similar to mine (and that of so many other readers), all I can ask is that you try to believe me when I say there is another way, and that change is possible.

We have nothing to be ashamed of. Nothing is wrong with us – and nothing ever was.

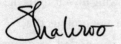

To find out more about behavioural change and creating healthy new habits, find me online @ShahrooIzadi or in 'The Last Diet Crew' Facebook group, a community for sharing and motivation. I'd love to hear from you and find out how your Last Diet journey is progressing.

shahroo_izadi
ShahrooIzadi
www.facebook.com/TheKindnessMethod

introduction

The last time you ever start from scratch again

I'm going to show you how to enjoyably manage your weight for the rest of your life, and I'll do it without telling you what to eat. Because, both from my personal experience of losing eight stone and through my professional experience of working in addiction treatment, I know that telling people how and why they should change is not effective. As a behavioural change specialist in private practice, I help people to achieve their weight-loss goals, whatever they may be, in whatever way best suits their bodies and lives.

I suspect you already know how to literally lose weight, and if you don't, then the briefest of Google searches will bring up all the nutritional information and dietary guidance you need to lose weight sensibly. The basic formulas for safe and effective weight management are widely available and our pool of effective diet options is growing every day.

So, if the problem isn't knowing what you need to do, or knowing how to do it, then why haven't you done it yet? These are the questions that this book is here to help you to answer, and your responses will enable you to create a weight-management plan that is specifically tailored to your needs. One that has your overall wellbeing in mind.

We often underestimate the amount of thought that is needed in order to create a truly sustainable default 'way of eating' for someone who has always struggled. We make the mistake of thinking that simply desire, desperation or visible results are enough to keep some people on track.

I imagine that the reason you bought this book is to understand why you even need it. I suspect it's not knowledge of a specific diet you're looking for, but self-knowledge. That's why, when it comes to helping plan the specifics of what you'll be eating or not eating to lose and maintain weight, I won't profess to know what choices are best for your body. Instead I will simply provide the guidance you need to draw out your own wisdom. *The Last Diet* needs you to get on board with the belief that, regardless of why you want to lose weight, how much you want to lose or what practical route you choose to take, your results won't be sustained in a meaningful way unless you commit to:

1. Liking yourself more every day

2. Getting to know yourself better every day

3. Believing in yourself more every day

People often believe that they'll only be capable of doing these things once they've reached a goal weight or size. Quite the opposite is true. Starting to be kinder to yourself immediately (regardless of your weight) will make weight-loss goals easier to achieve – although you may have to change your definition of what 'being kinder' means, but we'll come to that later. For many of you, redefining what 'kind decisions' are when it comes to our bodies will bring about the biggest shift in how you see weight loss.

I hope that one day, weight-loss books will simply be evidence-based updates of food and exercise guidance for those who want to literally lose fat from their bodies for whatever reason is important to them. Perhaps because they're prone to putting on weight easily, and they'd just prefer not to, for their own good reasons. As it stands however, almost all of the conversations I have with people about their struggles to shift unwanted weight feature themes like low self-esteem, negative body image and self-sabotage. Luckily though, things seem to be going in the right direction. People are starting to realise what I've seen to be the case over and over again: **believing you're entitled to be happy regardless of your size is actually what helps you to be a size you're happy with.**

So, with that in mind, The Last Diet is a kinder weight-loss plan, that focuses on written exercises designed to increase your self-esteem and self-awareness, not simply physical exercises designed to make you lose fat. This book will help you to design a long-term eating, exercise and wellbeing routine – on purpose. One with self-created guidelines that you're OK with following, even when it's difficult. Because it's much harder to rebel against your diet when you know you created it yourself, and that you put in a lot of work to make sure it's the one with your overall best interests at heart.

Although the word 'diet' gets a bad rap, it needn't only be associated with fads and miracle cures. Of *course* your diet will play a part in the process of you losing weight and keeping it off. The same way it will have played a part in you gaining weight or not being able to keep it off. Your diet is simply a description of things you consume. In this sense, you're always on a diet, it just may not be a predictable one, or one that you've chosen on purpose.

This book is for those who want to create their diet on purpose. Those who have come to realise that without some basic guidelines to follow, their current automatic eating habits will result in their bodies looking and feeling a way they're not happy with. Some people will conclude through the exploratory, preparatory exercises in this book that they can create broad, loose guidelines, while others will decide they need more specific ones.

Some people will never need a book like this. They can't understand how anyone would feel they need to follow self-imposed rules that keep them from enjoying the 'relatively harmless joy and comfort' that food is, whenever they like, and just 'knowing when to stop'. From my experience, these people tend to fall into one of these two categories. Some fall into both. I was always particularly jealous of those people:

1. People who can eat however and whatever they choose, and be content with how those choices make them look and feel

2. People who, regardless of what's going on in their lives, are able to make natural and spontaneous choices for their bodies that are in their best interests long term

You may find it impossible to imagine you could ever belong to one of these categories. But I truly that believe we all can, some of us just need extra help staying in them. I now consider myself to exist in one of those categories most of the time. That said, I still sometimes have to remember that I wasn't always one of those people, and that in order to avoid subtly gaining unwanted weight long term, I'll always need simple default eating guidelines to fall back on.

Throughout this book, I use examples from my own experience of struggling with losing weight and keeping it off. I also draw on the stories of clients I've met through my private practice and habit-change workshops. You will read jargon-free explanations of the approaches I learned working in addiction treatment; motivational concepts that I've seen change people's entire lives for the better. You'll understand why, as soon as I realised the same concepts work for weight loss, I became dedicated to telling everyone about them immediately.

In essence, if you learn the fundamentals of motivation and good planning, you will always feel equipped to understand and change unwanted habits that may emerge around food and exercise, for the rest of your life, without handing yourself over to an 'expert' who needs time to get to know you. The ultimate 'way of eating' you create during this process will eventually become your new normal. But maybe in five years your body or your routine will change, or life circumstances will mean that you can't stick to the same plan anymore. Or you just don't want to. If and when that happens, you can return to the exercises in this book to find everything you need to create a new plan that suits your needs.

For some people, losing weight using this book will be a very simple and practical process of planning things like food choices more consciously and making sure they stay motivated until their new habits can be trusted to their autopilot. Their inability to maintain the weight they want isn't caused by anything much deeper than what they eat and how much they do or don't move around; in other words, their unwanted eating habits aren't wrapped up in strong emotional needs, current or historical. Perhaps they simply associate food with fuel, joy and comfort, but some of the food types and quantities they eat happen to be making them gain or maintain unwanted weight. Perhaps they don't believe any of their value lies in whether they are slim. But it's of course still their prerogative to look how they like, and they just happen to want to be slimmer. Maybe they've never needed to diet in the past but their bodies just aren't playing ball with the status quo anymore.

I was never one of these people. The way I'm made up physically means I've always naturally gained weight very quickly. Still, I always knew that staying overweight was largely due to what I ate, and most importantly why and how I ate it. How much I moved around played a part too, but not such a big one. Throughout my life, there have been a number of reasons why I have eaten in ways that make me gain weight, ranging from:

- Frequent snacking and bingeing on large quantities of unquestionably fattening foods in an attempt to relieve anxiety, stress and low mood

- Loving fattening foods and finding them extremely comforting

- Unconsciously wanting to stay overweight

- Yo-yo dieting and extended bingeing in response to falling off track with restrictive plans

- A childhood spent scheming to get my hands on forbidden 'fattening' foods

- Abusing food to relieve myself from the realisation that I was abusing food

- Never establishing what a healthy, 'normal' way to eat was for my body

How it works

You will use the guidance provided in this book to create a 'normal' way to eat that suits your needs, based on undisputed, common sense principles. Regardless of your current eating style, this process includes the elements we can all agree are a good idea in the short and long term, like:

- Staying hydrated

- Eating vegetables

- Not staying hungry for long

- Eating a variety of foods

- Eating mindfully and enjoying the process of eating

- Not consuming large amounts of sugar

- Not eating in ways that make you feel anxious or in a low mood

- Not eating in ways that make you feel tired or sluggish

- Not eating compulsively

- Eating in ways that give you sustained energy as opposed to a quick 'hit'

- Eating in ways that help you feel focused and energetic

- Eating in ways that give your body a sense of true nourishment

Essentially, The Last Diet is an opportunity to learn how to make choices for your body and mind that you'd want a loved one to make for theirs. That is the most important habit you will develop during this entire process, and one that will make it most meaningful across every area of your life, as well as helping you to achieve your weight-loss goals.

my story

I know you because I am you

The Last Diet was created largely from my experience in two main areas:

1. A lifelong struggle with my weight

2. A career in addiction treatment

There's no denying it, I was a chubby baby. At some point in my childhood, I started realising that my body was causing concern to those around me. When I was around nine years old, my mother began worrying that my weight was becoming an issue. So she started changing what she cooked at home and drawing my attention to the things I ate that I shouldn't eat so much of. She didn't tell me outright that it was because those foods were causing me to gain weight and that gaining weight was a bad thing. And, as a child, I simply picked up on the fact that there was now a new way to be 'good' or 'bad'. This was the first time I realised that some foods were naughty and that eating them would make people unhappy with me.

I had already started to suspect something was up. I remember kids in junior school asking me why I was bigger than them. I remember being in a school uniform shop once when I was about ten and the shop assistant telling my mum that the sizes didn't go up any higher, and that she'd have to start altering my skirts. My mum then started to sew extra panels into the side and, when I went to school, I realised that parts of my skirt were a very slightly different shade to other girls'.

As I became more aware that there was something 'wrong' with me, I became more dependent on behaviours like bingeing and secret eating that would cause me to gain a lot of weight very quickly. As soon as I had a chance to consume the foods that my mother had controlled at home to slow down my weight gain, I would eat them like there was no tomorrow. I would obsess over getting my hands on them and strategise to ensure I could be alone with them. I would lie about how much of them I had eaten. I'm not proud to admit the lengths I'd go to for 'hit' of the forbidden foods. And it was very much a hit, because that's the other force that was embedding my dependency on the forbidden foods: they were very high in sugar and fat. Food addiction was a very real part of my life before I understood what it was or indeed that it even existed.

In a similar way to what happens with many drugs, my tolerance grew and eventually I needed more of those hits more frequently to get my fix. As a result, I continued to gain weight at a rapid pace. By the time I was about twelve, the GP was telling me I was obese, and I had already grown very accustomed to being told by my peers that I was fat (and that being fat was a bad thing).

During secondary school, I started believing that boys didn't fancy fat girls and fat girls aren't popular unless they're funny or have something else to bring to the table. These assumptions began to turn into a self-fulfilling belief, where for example I would choose to stay at home and binge instead of going to a party, because I decided that while I was fat, I wasn't going to have much fun. TV shows and movies didn't help either. It seemed to be a very common storyline that it wasn't until someone lost weight that they became desirable, popular and self-respecting.

Both my relationship with food and with my weight started to become a problem I desperately wanted to deal with. I went to my mum asking for help and, with the best intentions in the world, she started calling for back up. She approached the issue from every angle you could think of. Anything to stop me crying when I'd come home and say someone had made fun of me at school. We'd go to nutritionists, slimming clubs, dieticians, herbalists, hormone specialists and hypnotists. We came at the problem from two angles:

1. Find out what's wrong with my body

2. Find out how not to be fat anymore

My mum would sit there and explain (what she thought was) the whole story to the 'experts' over and over again. What she didn't know was that at this stage I wasn't sure whether it was my secret binges on the forbidden foods that was the issue or if it was a problem with the way my body was working. By this point, I wasn't aware of how much I was already using food as a drug to help me cope with all the social, physical and emotional discomforts of being overweight. Since so many of my impulsive, rebellious, opportunistic eating habits had developed in secret, I didn't register how my actions were spiralling. Plus, I was just a kid!

During the initial consultations and assessments, I was made very aware of how long my weight had been causing concern. I witnessed countless pitches from experts who I realise now could only sell my mum a fix if they concluded that I needed fixing. I became more and more conscious that something was the matter with me and that it was costing those around me time, money and energy to try to fix it (however hard they tried to hide this fact from me). Behind every consultation room door was a new person who would weigh me, prod me, confirm something was wrong with me and offer me a cure.

As a result of many of these appointments, I would adopt various 'expert-recommended' crash diets, and I genuinely wanted them to change my body and my life. But of course, they never did, because every time I fell off the wagon, I would binge. By my mid-teens, I seriously didn't want to be overweight anymore and was prepared to do anything to make that possible. Plus, my mum and I were a team, and although she never put pressure on me, she knew the rules I was meant to be following for each different attempt. Quite naturally, she was disappointed when I couldn't keep up the plans because she knew how desperately I wanted to be slimmer. The problem was that she couldn't really be the team mate she wanted to be because she didn't know the level my dependence on food had reached. Even if I'd wanted to, I didn't have anywhere near enough insight or self-awareness to explain what was going on for me.

So, over and over again I'd fall off track with these plans, become disillusioned and end up heavier than when I started. Any success they brought eventually became a curse, because the diets that gave me quick transformations were the ones I couldn't sustain, the ones that made life miserable. People would applaud me when I was visibly smaller, but they would notice every time I gained weight too. This of course made me feel self-conscious and afraid of being judged, as well as fostering the belief that people preferred me when I wasn't fat.

I reinforced this belief throughout my life, associating not being able to manage my weight with disappointments in other areas. I would look for evidence to confirm my suspicion that being fat was bad. And of course, growing up in the nineties as a girl in the Western world, there was a lot of it flying around.

Since my eating habits became entirely associated with my weight from such a young age, from birth to the time I went to university to study psychology, my 'way of eating' had looked like this:

- Breast milk

- Food my mum knew was healthy for kids in general

- Food my mum knew would help me lose weight + secret binges

- Extreme diet plans

- Extreme diet plans + secret binges

- Food my mum knew would help me lose weight + secret binges

- Extreme diet plans

- Extreme diet plans + secret binges

- Etc.

When my parents dropped me off on campus to live on my own for the first time at university, I was already close to being my heaviest ever. However, I had decided that I would transform while I was there, eventually, by starving myself. And so in the meantime I would eat whatever I wanted, whenever I wanted, however I wanted for the first time in my life. And oh boy, did I go for it. In that first term of university I ate in a way that caused me to gain a lot more weight. I also developed a regular weed smoking habit that didn't help matters. It was a disastrous marriage of substances, joining together to help me avoid and delay emotional discomfort as well as making me want to eat more.

As I grew closer to some of my friends at university, I discovered that they had a very different relationship with food than I did. When we went to the supermarket, they knew which ingredients to buy in order to cook a number of meals that were part of their ordinary way of eating. I, on the other hand, was leaving with shopping bags full of either celery and seeds or chips and trifles. I didn't have a dozen 'meals' in mind because my meals had always consisted of things my mum had cooked and things that were forbidden. Both for cultural reasons and the fact my mum reigned over the kitchen in my house, the only meals I ate regularly were either way too complicated for me to want to learn how to cook, or way too 'healthy' for me to be convinced to cook. A 'big shop' for me often involved picking what I wanted to eat that day and just multiplying it by fourteen to last me two weeks.

I carried on like this into my second year of university, until I got to a point where I was used to waking up feeling lethargic and heavy. It's lucky I wasn't interested in alcohol at that time, as I imagine that would have made the situation much worse. During this time there were of course still attempts to lose weight. Although I told my mum that I was done with all the expert outsourcing, I was still determined to one day be slim. After all, my flawed belief system told me that it wasn't until I had lost weight that I could really go out, take up the space I deserve to and enjoy my life.

I'd got to a stage where if I caught myself starting to feel good or enjoy myself for whatever reason, I would immediately think 'this would be so much better if I wasn't still fat'. Often, I would catch a glimpse of myself and not only realise that I had expanded but also that I had stopped taking pride in my appearance and my surroundings. So, in response, I would punish myself by deciding to embark on another crash diet and life transformation plan. These would commence between one and five times a week, and last for anything between one hour and six weeks. But now they were harder to keep to than when I lived at home, since I didn't have a routine or any supervision. Plus, my addictive eating patterns had a hold on me that made the withdrawals really painful whenever I'd try to rashly deprive myself, thinking that's what I deserved for letting things get to this stage.

I was also able to adopt much more extreme diets, ones that my mum would understandably never have allowed. I started abusing laxatives and taking appetite suppressants from the internet that were essentially amphetamines. I could go days without eating if

I wanted to, without anyone noticing. So not only was university a fertile ground for my food addiction to spiral, it was also the perfect place for my quick-fix, all-or-nothing, lose weight at any cost thinking to get worse.

I even very briefly had a gastric band fitted in secret. That threw into the mix a lot of fear, shame, vomiting, pain and medical complications.

Plus it didn't fix anything – aside from the fact it obviously did nothing to address my relationship with food, the kinds of foods I'd always binged on were 'soft' and could pass through the band anyway.

Whilst the procedure itself may have been completely reversible, the process was psychologically scarring. I was left feeling more hopeless than ever and so isolated in my sadness. It was only very recently that I've been able to talk about it without getting upset.

You'd think that an experience like that would have made me take it easier on my body, but quite the opposite was true. As soon as the band got taken out, I got straight back on the yo-yo wagon. The realization that even such an extreme intervention couldn't 'work' on me made me want to punish my body even more. That said, the lengths I showed myself I was prepared to go to alone also reminded me of how desperately I wanted to change. So, I kept signing up for new diets and pills and miracle cures.

On one occasion, I continued long after the usual six weeks, and although I used a combination of very unhealthy methods, I managed to lose a lot of weight. I went from a size 20 to a size 8. For the first time in my entire life, I was undeniably thin.

So, I lived as a thin person for a couple of years during my last year of university and the year following it. My hair was thinning and I struggled to focus, but I didn't care because for the first time

I was *thin*. Although you will have gathered that this story doesn't end well, I have to admit that it was all that I'd hoped it would be in a lot of ways, but largely because I'd spent my life treating it as the criterion I needed to meet in order to enjoy myself.

I wore the clothes I'd always dreamt of wearing; I went on a holiday and wore a bikini the whole time; I stood up straight and acted more spontaneously. Plus, the world applauded me. And not just because of my achievement, because I was thin. I wish this wasn't true but it was. I knew this because coming into contact with new people as a slim person was an entirely different experience. The suspicions I'd had that fat people weren't treated as well as thin people – at least in the UK – were confirmed. When I met people for the first time as a slim person and told them how much weight I'd lost, they usually reacted to my 'before' pictures with shock and horror. 'That doesn't even look like you!', 'Wow, what an achievement, you looked ten years older then!', 'You look SO much better now', 'Make sure you keep up the good work!', 'It just suits your face more to be thin', 'Boys must be queuing up now . . .' I lapped it up.

Then there were the people who knew and cared for me, who communicated their relief that I was finally thin. They treated my weight loss as a done deal, a solution to a problem that had been low-key concerning everyone for a while, not least because of how much it concerned me. Everything was fixed as far as other people were concerned, and I deserved praise, so they were happy to tell me how much better I looked.

But it wasn't a fix. They didn't know that I hadn't found a long-term solution to staying slim other than things like skipping meals, white knuckling it and abusing appetite suppressants. Plus, every time someone told me how much better I looked now, it made me think they didn't think I looked fine before. Nonetheless, in the short term at least, people reacting positively to my weight loss spurred me on.

Predictably, the combination of not knowing what to eat to maintain my new size and needing constant external validation meant that once the compliments died down and it turned out that all life's problems hadn't disappeared, I subtly started lapsing. I ate to deal with the disappointment of slimness not being the solution to my low self-esteem and also because I was starving all the time. I slipped back into old ways – in that I slipped back into no 'ways', just impulsive, isolated binges – and my weight crept back on until, before I knew it, I wasn't thin anymore. It was like it had all been a dream. I was back where I started and, although it made me desperately sad and disillusioned, it was also strangely comforting in its familiarity and predictability.

Over the next few years, well into my late twenties, I repeated this pattern of losing huge amounts of weight at rapid speeds once I'd hit another 'rock bottom' and then gaining it again. Many had learned to stop commenting on my always fluctuating weight. As an old colleague once said when I walked into a meeting after four months of not seeing her, 'Oh you're thin again! We were all just debating whether we thought you'd be thin or not this time.' I'd say that between the ages of 23 and 30, I spent 20 per cent of the time very slim, 60 per cent very overweight and the other 20 per cent in the transition process.

By this time, I had started living in London. I got my master's degree and when it came to choosing an area of psychology to specialise in, I chose addiction. I started with an unpaid, one-year placement in an NHS service in north-west London, where I was introduced to the world of addiction treatment for the first time. Admittedly, when I walked into the waiting room on the first day for my induction, I remember wondering whether a placement somewhere like this was really going to be worth working two side-jobs for. But just hours into my job there, I knew I'd found my career path for life.

Day after day, I witnessed people's entire lives transform thanks to the help they were getting from my colleagues. I grew obsessed, and gave my role more time and energy than I'd ever given any paid role before. I wanted to learn as much as I could. I soon figured out that one of the best ways to learn was to work on the reception desk. This way I could speak to the patients, hear their stories, help them with forms and make them tea. I learned how to really listen to people and make them feel heard.

As the months passed and my obsession with my role grew evident to my colleagues, I started being given more responsibility. By the end of my placement I was confident that I could go straight into a paid addiction worker role, and that's what I did. My new job was to assess and treat drug addicts using a range of the latest motivational tools, which I was continuously trained in. In contrast to the NHS placement, I was no longer in clinical environments, so most of the approaches I used were focused on motivational exercises, talking therapies and support groups as opposed to prescriptions and risk assessments.

I kept working my way up in the field until eventually I became a consultant and trainer, advising healthcare organisations on the best approaches to use in addiction treatment.

I became knowledgeable in new approaches I had never heard of, and built on what I already knew from my first-hand experience and previous training. I started to travel across the country delivering training to clinical, community and prison staff teams, all of whom wanted additional tools to help them motivate their complex and resistant clients to make lasting changes that they could sustain independently.

The training I delivered would include a lot of written exercises that delegates could try out so that they felt comfortable going back and using them with their own clients. I would mainly guide them to complete 'maps'. This simply involved writing a theme in the middle of a page and scattering ideas around it, as opposed to writing things in a list. In the first few months of delivering training, I'd ask delegates to populate their maps using examples from one of their client's lives. But something kept happening that made me tweak this: people wanted to complete the maps using examples from their own lives, to use the motivational and planning exercises to explore their own unwanted habits. This didn't surprise me, as seeing how effective these tools were at work, I'd also begun to re-approach the ever-looming task of losing weight with more focus on my motivation and personal development.

Although the maps helped me to gain more insight into my behaviours and lose a bit of weight by decreasing the frequency and severity of my binges, I still didn't have a 'way of eating'. I knew from my work across addiction that meaningful change had to be realistic and enjoyable. But I had no idea how to sustain a way of eating that managed my weight and was all of these things at the same time. That's were OA came in.

OA, or Overeaters Anonymous, is a twelve-step programme for people who feel that their behaviours around food have become unmanageable. I came across it when I was doing research for a client on what free support was available. Of course, I had heard of the Alcoholics Anonymous programme, but in order for that to be effective you have to abstain from alcohol entirely. You can't be abstinent from food entirely.

I went to check out OA and learned that some of the same concepts that help us stop doing something altogether can also help us to keep doing it, but differently. I learned that although everyone at OA followed a prescribed twelve-step programme, when it came to the food guidelines they had to follow to be in a state of recovery, everyone's were different. There seemed to be some common themes that ran through people's individual programmes – like trying not to eat refined sugar or starchy carbs, and of course going through the required personal development exercises. But for most, when it came to food, they had different definitions of what lapse and relapse looked like, based on their bodies, their goals and their experience.

Over time, I combined my learning from OA, clinical addiction treatment and training feedback to create an entire personal development plan that enabled me to lose weight gradually, meaningfully and more enjoyably than ever before. I created new maps that focused more on my self-esteem and I designed exercises that helped me find sensible personal definitions for words like 'healthy' and 'moderation'. I kept the weight off this time because I finally realised that there was never anything wrong with me, I just never had the tools, self-awareness or self-belief I needed to make lasting changes.

The Last Diet is a collection of all the tools and knowledge I needed, in the format I needed it, to finally change. It's the book I wish I had twenty years ago.

your story

You're the expert

The Last Diet will give you the tools and guidance you need to write all the next chapters of your story when it comes to how you treat your body.

Regardless of whether you've spent a lifetime struggling to manage your weight or just the past few months, the exercises in this book will enable you to design a plan of change that is most suited to your needs specifically. For them to be effective, however, it's important that you commit to completing them comprehensively and with complete honesty. You should feel that you are taking a much deeper, more exploratory look at what works for you and what habits have brought you to where you are today. Although it will be difficult at times to write down things about your current or previous habits that you're not proud of, this is precisely the kind of investment it's important to make in this process.

When it comes to recording the reasons you want to lose weight, don't worry about what you think you should write: just write what's true. No one will judge you; you're allowed to have whatever motivators you like. Plus, when it comes to gaining momentum in the early stages of change, it's very much a case of 'whatever gets you there'. So if, like me, when you're really honest about what's likely to get you out of bed on a rainy morning to exercise, it's something like 'the thought of feeling great in my favourite jeans as opposed to 'the thought of not getting diabetes', then that's OK. You will find that The Last Diet is not a process of finding yourself, but rather, a process of meeting yourself, and being fine with whoever you meet.

In this book I am going to guide you to the point where you can draw out your own wisdom. I will give you a basic framework in which you can establish and create your own ideal conditions for success.

When I began writing *The Last Diet*, one of the first things I considered was who I was trying to help, and how I could help as many people as possible. So I started by thinking about what we – all of us who have struggled to maintain our weight, whatever the reason – have in common. I scrolled through pages and pages of client notes, and I saw that despite having vastly different stories, those who wanted to lose weight were often saying quite similar things when it came to the changes they wanted to make. I created a top twenty list and, from that, have assumed in writing *The Last Diet* that some or all of these things are true for you:

1. You're tired of making the same resolutions every year (or every Monday)

2. You create meticulous weight-loss plans but can't seem to keep them up

3. You're confused as to why you can't stop behaving a certain way around food, even though you really want to and have all the information you need

4. You feel demoralised and disillusioned after a series of unsuccessful attempts to change

5. You're tired of signing up to miracle plans and quick-fix solutions that aren't sustainable

6. The way you tend to speak to yourself when it comes to weight loss is unkind and self-sabotaging

7. You feel as though you're living life on hold, waiting to achieve your weight-loss goals

8. You believe you'll always be an all-or-nothing person with an 'addictive personality'

9. Your inability to manage your weight is negatively impacting your relationships, social life, professional development or general wellbeing

10. You don't feel you have the self-esteem or self-belief needed to change

11. You struggle to adopt sensible weight-loss plans because slow progress doesn't keep you motivated

12. You're tired of declaring to loved ones that you're making changes, only to have to update them that you've once again fallen off the wagon

13. You want to set your own goals and create habits that fit into your lifestyle, based on what's important to you

14. Your body has changed and so the same weight-management methods that worked before aren't as effective

15. You want to explore healthier ways to deal with stress, worry and boredom than food and/or compulsive eating habits

16. You want to invest in personal development to become more self-aware in general about how you're treating yourself

17. You want to be able to keep your long-term weight-loss goals in mind instead of giving in to immediate temptation when it comes to food choices

18. You feel you don't have an 'off switch' when it comes to engaging in unwanted habits around food

19. You've never found a long-term 'healthy' way of eating that enables you to freely enjoy food and also manage your weight

20. You think you lack the willpower to keep up a plan of change around eating

How your thinking patterns and general behaviours towards your body have developed over time may not be something you stop to consider very often. We're all always engaging in habits, and some will be autopilot ones. Through this process you may well realise that your current 'programming' of autopilot thoughts and behaviours has been influenced by external forces throughout your life; ones you haven't ever stopped to question.

You will continue to eat for the rest of your life whether you give it any thought or you don't. So why not choose to consider it, so that you have more say in the decisions you make instead of being led by self-defeating, unhelpful and unkind beliefs quite possibly carried over from childhood?

If you're a 'quick-fix' kind of person like me, you'll be happy to know you can go through the exercises in this book as quickly as you want and start making positive changes straight away. You can work your own way through to the action plan towards the end and start seeing the visible results soon after. You don't have to wait to book a session with me, turn up for a support group or part with another penny. Plus, the exercises you complete during this process will be ones you can come back to for the rest of your life, as part of a long-term commitment to checking in with yourself and making sure you feel happy about your relationship with food – and with yourself.

In my private practice, I've worked with many clients who have completely changed their relationships with food by using the methods in this book. People who had spent their entire lives never quite finding a way of eating that suits them. People who were demoralised and had lost hope of ever being truly happy with their bodies. People who had lost all the weight they wanted to, only to realise that nothing else in their life had improved at all – a realisation that was making them put the weight back on quickly. They used The Last Diet to take control of their story. And now, so will you.

the last diet

What it's all about

What is it?

The Last Diet is a weight-management programme that takes a deeper approach to changing unwanted eating habits. It's inspired by the motivational approaches that work in drug addiction treatment.

How is it different to other diets?

Instead of just focusing on food and exercise, The Last Diet also considers the self-esteem, self-awareness and self-belief you'll need to sustain your results enjoyably and meaningfully in the long term. Choosing what you eat to lose and to manage your weight will be entirely up to you. I will help you access the information you need to create the plans and goals that are best for you. But I won't presume to know what's best for your body.

The Last Diet assumes that you pretty much know how to lose weight already, but that you need more help understanding why you can't get going or stick to your eating or exercising plan even though you want to.

What will I have to do?

First, you'll work through this book, completing written exercises that I guide you through in order. These are designed to best prepare you for the changes ahead. As soon as you've completed your first written exercise at the end of the next chapter, you can consider yourself 'on' The Last Diet.

Then, when you've finished reading this book, you'll officially activate the more practical eating and exercise elements of your desired weight-loss plan.

(Just in case you're thinking, 'That means I have plenty of time for some last blowouts first', then for now, just try to observe that thought process. Curiously question how much sense it makes. And I don't say this as a professional habit expert, but as a professional excuse-maker.)

Are the exercises hard work?

They're simple to understand and to complete, but they're intended to make you think hard, and in new ways. The intention is that you use the process of reading this book as the first in many opportunities you will now be taking to put time aside for yourself and invest in your wellbeing.

If an exercise in this book requires you to think back to previous failed attempts, for example, it's absolutely worth your time to jog your memory in every way you can. If that means rooting through old calendars and diaries, finding old subscription emails or just taking fifteen extra minutes to sit in silence and really cast your mind back, then it's important that you do it – even if revisiting past failures feels uncomfortable at times. The harder you work on the written exercises, the easier it will feel when it comes to practically changing your eating habits in everyday settings. They need to feel like an investment, to make you feel more accountable and also that you're making truly informed decisions when it comes to creating your bespoke plan of change.

I assume that in buying this book you're acknowledging that it's actually becoming hard work to stay the way you are. If you're anything like I used to be, you're probably spending most of your energy beating yourself up for not having changed yet. I can assure you that none of the exercises in this book are as hard as that.

What's with the maps?

I'll be asking you to complete simple mind maps throughout this process. I have found that it can be very effective to have different thoughts and observations scattered around a page, as opposed to written out as a list. Well populated maps can provide a crucial snapshot of collective ideas, and represent something visually that it is incredibly difficult to recall all at once in our heads, especially when we're feeling like throwing in the towel.

As you work through each chapter, you'll see that some maps will prove useful across all areas of your life, whereas others are only applicable to the specific habits you're focused on changing at that time. When you've completed all the maps in this book, you will have a wealth of visual resources to hand, designed to boost your self-esteem, self-belief and self-awareness.

What's with all the mentions of kindness?

I believe that we all know what kindness looks and feels like, in the context of our relationships with others, both when it comes to giving and receiving it. It's great. The problem is that we're often not very kind to ourselves. And, as I've seen so many times through my work and personal experience, it is those who struggle to be kind to themselves who have the hardest time when they try to make lasting, meaningful changes to their eating habits.

So, what is kindness? A thesaurus search brings up synonyms such as: patience, understanding, consideration, compassion and helpfulness. The Last Diet approach is based on the belief that if we commit to behaving in these ways towards our bodies across every possible area of our lives, then our food choices will follow suit with less effort.

What if my version of kindness is eating chocolate and chips for dinner every night?

In this process you will learn that although kindness is about being gentle with ourselves and enjoying our lives as much as possible overall, when it comes to making difficult changes kindness also means choosing to put ourselves in some manageable short-term discomfort to achieve our most valued goals. It means believing in our ability to do difficult things and challenge our own self-limiting beliefs.

The Last Diet helps you shift your definition of kind behaviours away from being habits that give you instant relief, comfort or distraction, to choices you'll be glad you made for yourself the next day. In many cases, riding out a short-term urge or craving isn't an act of unkindness or depriving yourself, it's an opportunity to show yourself how capable you are. Plus, it's a necessary step to take as many times as possible if the craving is to become less powerful in the long term.

In order to help you act more kindly, this process will require you to first *think* more kindly and not treat it as a punishment or remedy. I've seen many clients fall off track with their plans by thinking that depriving themselves of the things that turn down the volume on unwelcome internal chatter in the short term is a punishment. Often a lapse is prompted by the internal message: 'Its unkind to deprive myself of things that comfort me.' In order to get to where you want to be using The Last Diet, you need to be OK with curiously and consciously listening to your self-sabotaging thoughts and willingly feeling your impulses, instead of impulsively acting on them or pushing them to the back of your mind as soon as they pop up.

If at any point in this process you're unsure about whether the choices you make for your body are kind or not, simply consider whether they're the same choices you'd make for the body of the person you love most in the world.

How will I know what to actually eat?

When you get to the practical planning stages of this book I will ask you to complete a very comprehensive enquiry into what foods and ways of eating are best for you and your body specifically.

Will I have to keep coming back to this book to keep up my results?

Although I will encourage you to reflect on your progress by looking at your maps and taking a keen lifelong interest in your personal development, you will feel progressively less dependent on the written guidance and tools in this book over time. That's because:

- You'll have 'time under your belt' and enjoy results that you'll want to protect and sustain

- You'll have overcome challenging situations that demonstrate how capable you are. This will make you want to keep surprising yourself

- You'll be able to quickly remember why it's important for you to stay on track. This will help you to waste less time entertaining any unhelpful excuses to lapse

- You'll develop a new set of automatic behaviours. Realising you can choose them when it comes to eating habits will get you excited about what other kind habits you can choose for yourself

- The exercises will have helped to increase your self-esteem in an authentic way, so that you don't associate your worth with your weight, and therefore don't fall into the trap of throwing in the towel at the times when your weight invariably plateaus or fluctuates

- You will be less convinced by your own justifications to go off track. The more you practise noticing and questioning them, the less compelling they will become

- The generally kinder landscape of your life will be less accommodating to unkind eating habits

What kinds of people see the best results?

Those who:

- Invest time in getting really clear on why they want to change

- Understand why they haven't changed already

- Change for their own reasons

- Are prepared to own what works for them, even if it means they have to defend it to other people sometimes

- Are completely honest with themselves about why they want to change

- Expect their drive to waver from minute to minute for a while, and put strategies in place to ensure they stay on track when it inevitably dips

- Find a definition for kindness around their eating habits that has their best interests at heart across their entire lives

What beliefs do I need get on board with?

1. You're fine as you are

In order to lose weight with The Last Diet, you're going to have to start believing (or at least wanting to believe) that your body is worthy of kindness regardless of your weight. The process of losing weight will be much easier if you start trying to do all the things you plan to do when you've lost weight as soon as possible. Your weight may well fluctuate throughout your life for a range of reasons. It cannot be a criterion for liking yourself or enjoying your life.

2. Tough love isn't helpful

The Last Diet approach believes that tough love, warnings and scare tactics might get us going initially, but they don't keep us going. To keep pushing through and making kind choices for ourselves in those moments when it's most difficult, we need to focus on what we're moving towards, not what we're moving away from. We need to be given encouragement and positive feedback. Any tough love you think would actually be helpful for you is the kind you can give yourself through the initial exercises in this book.

3. Thoughts and feelings don't have to become actions

When it comes to our eating habits, even when our actions seem impulsive and on autopilot, we are still making a choice to follow our own commands. In order for The Last Diet to be most effective, you need to be willing to slow down your actions and curiously question the thoughts and feelings that drive them. You will need to develop a belief that urges and cravings are 'yoo-hoos' not 'YOU DO . . .'s. They are alerts, not commands.

4. Mental health is physical health

The Last Diet requires you to make your emotional wellbeing and personal development a priority. Not only because poor mental health can negatively impact your ability to take care of your physical health, but also because you may well discover during this process that your current unwanted eating habits are serving as short-term coping strategies for things like stress and anxiety.

5. Rock bottom isn't a prerequisite for change

Many traditional addiction treatment approaches believe that people don't change until things have become truly unbearable. For some, this is the case. I've met people who remember the moment they decided to change their habits and immediately did so without ever looking back.

Most of the time, however, especially when it comes to more day-to-day habits, it's not unusual to have loads of 'rock bottoms'. I can't count the number of times I cried in a changing room where nothing fit me (again) thinking, 'That's it, I never thought things would get this bad. Things are changing TODAY.' Yet despite this, my rock bottoms gradually just kept getting lower, and I eventually normalised them. This was especially the case when it came to numbers on scales.

6. Forewarned is forearmed

Many of us have made the mistake of thinking our desire to change is enough to get us there. As a result, when it comes to creating a plan of action for weight loss, we immediately turn our attention to what we'll eat or not eat. We assume that simply knowing what to do and knowing we want to do it is enough to achieve our goals.

The Last Diet believes that in order to gain momentum with weight loss and maintain it long term, we need to do some far less obvious planning than meal plans and grocery lists. When it comes to ingrained patterns, any change from the status quo can bring physical cravings and urges as well as emotional discomfort, so we need to have a plan for how we'll respond to internal and external triggers. Even if our plan is to do nothing, but on purpose.

Is there anything I won't be allowed to eat again?

No.

that's it

A snapshot of reasons to change

The written exercise at the end of this chapter will mark the first step in starting your Last Diet, and the last time you'll feel you're 'starting from scratch' again. Because this time your goals will be built on foundations of self-knowledge, self-belief and self-care. The plans for change you have tried before probably focused on what foods to eat, how regularly to exercise, what measurements to take, etc. This time will be different. This time you'll work on how you think, act and speak towards yourself before you even consider how you'll eat! And in so doing, you will develop an arsenal of assets and tools that will anchor you and enable you to top up your motivation levels again and again, in a way that simple meal plans and numbers on scales just don't.

Much of the inspiration for the exercises in this chapter came from my time working in substance misuse treatment. In many of the community services I was placed at, there was often a drop-in service, where people could walk in off the street and ask for help. A lot of the time, they would (understandably) expect to be able to speak to someone and get help straight away. Unfortunately, however, this was rarely the case. Due to a shortage of resources, most people could only be assessed that day, and then given a time to return days or weeks later when they could start sessions with a keyworker or attend a support group. Over and over, I would see people for whom things had come to a head walk through the door ready to make changes, only to be told they couldn't start yet.

Very often their decision to come in was a direct result of a 'rock bottom'. Perhaps their addiction had caused them go to lengths they never dreamed they would, or an incident had taken place that shocked them and brought to their attention how important it had become to change. Perhaps they'd finally got to a tipping point where they truly believed in that moment that the negatives of their actions outweighed the positives.

Often people walked in with a sense of urgency. It felt as though they had got to that moment that so many of us do after resolving to make the same changes over and over again: feeling fed up, out of control and ready to do whatever it takes to change the status quo. While this is actually the opposite of the attitude and perspective this book will encourage you to adopt in order to stay motivated in the long run, it's very useful for getting going. In these moments, we have naturally achieved the state that the early exercises in this book are designed to bring about – but in a more meaningful, positive and sustained way. Sometimes when we hit a 'rock bottom', we briefly and organically stumble upon:

- Belief that it's incredibly important and urgent to change the status quo (because of all the negative impacts)

- Belief in our ability to change the status quo (because of our desperation to do so or because we haven't experienced withdrawals yet)

These moments can be absolutely golden when it comes to finding the drive to get us going, but they are often fleeting and temporary. That's why it was so frustrating to see addicts coming in to the drop-in session for help when they'd reached this point but not be able to grasp the opportunity there and then.

What would often happen is that people wouldn't turn up for the future appointment they'd been given. Of course, this could be for a number of reasons, but when I called them to ask why they hadn't come back and try to make another appointment with them, they often sounded considerably less concerned than they did that first time, and definitely less motivated to do something about their unwanted habits. Time had passed and perhaps some of the negative impacts had become more manageable. Bodies had recovered to some extent and levels of desperation to change had decreased. This put me in a tricky position: on the one hand I was happy to hear that things didn't sound as bad as they did before. On the other hand, a big part of me wanted to remind the person on the phone of how bad they told me it had got and all the reasons why it was likely that it would get that bad – or worse – again, if they didn't address their legitimate concerns about their behaviours.

I wanted to warn them, essentially. To stop them from forgetting, to relay back what they'd told me before. To ask them what they thought would be different this time and what made them think everything would be OK, even if they kept repeating the same patterns over and over again. But I couldn't. Partly because good practitioners know that trying to 'save' people doesn't do them any favours. And partly because I knew from my experience with my weight and body struggles that if someone decided it was their job to remind me of what I should be doing and what's best for me, I'd become defensive, and feel more inclined to engage in the behaviours that made things worse (I would eat to distract from anger and annoyance and to demonstrate that I can do whatever the hell I like with my body). Plus, I would always assume that they had misunderstood my needs and struggles.

I'd spent a few months witnessing people come in to drug treatment services ready to change and then not coming back, when a colleague from another drug service taught me something they had implemented that was really helping. When people came in asking for help, as well as assessing them, practitioners asked them to write themselves a little note, in their own handwriting, that gave a snapshot of why they had chosen to come in to ask for help. Then, if they didn't come back for a second appointment, the service would post that note to them. This meant that people would be presented with something they couldn't push back against: a snapshot of themselves, by themselves and for themselves.

This small change had made a huge difference to how many people decided to come back and ask for help again. And the great thing was, they didn't need to feel as awful as they did on that first day to want to come back, they just needed to remember how bad things had been. Often they could recognise that what they had written to themselves was a description of the kind of day that was becoming more and more frequent, even if it wasn't how they felt the day they received it.

The exercise you will complete in this chapter will help you to capture those same moments: the ones when it's clear to you why it's important for you to change. It's an opportunity to write all the negatives in one place and show yourself that although motivation and importance will waver from day to day, overall, the negatives are outweighing the positives and you do want to change.

Things will present themselves every single day that will make you minimise, trivialise and normalise the behaviours that on other days come together and make things feel unmanageable and out of control. For example, when I was trying to lose weight, I could often trace a binge back to an experience of deciding that my goals weren't important in that moment. This could be something like a great evening out with friends a few weeks into a weight-loss diet, eating whatever I liked and genuinely enjoying myself. The next day I'd wake up and my all-or-nothing thinking patterns would mean all I could do was fixate on all the other things I wished I could eat since I'd already been so 'bad.'

Trivialising overeating, bingeing and eating mindlessly over and over again would always leave me in the same place: more unhappy in how my body felt and looked. In that moment, when I would tell myself that I should have fun and treat food like a joy, I wasn't able to remember that I didn't know how to do that yet, for one reason or another, even if other people could. I couldn't (and didn't want to) recall all the times I hadn't managed to do it before when the circumstances had been identical. I couldn't (and didn't want to) focus my attention on how I'd feel in a day or week, when history would dictate that I'd still be in a cycle of bingeing and self-loathing. I told myself I was 'living in the moment' and 'eating intuitively'. In theory of course, this is great. It's how I live now much of the time. But it's something that, for people like me, needs to be learned and practised and understood. I couldn't wing it yet.

Another method of trivialising my desire to lose weight was by berating myself about how silly my problems were compared to those of others. Working in substance misuse treatment, this wasn't difficult to do. I would meet people who had problems I couldn't even imagine dealing with. I heard accounts of extreme trauma and abuse. I saw people's immense gratitude for things I took for granted every day. Then I would go home at the end of the day (usually hungry and tired) and when it came to trying not to order a take-out, I'd think, 'Who cares about my weight? I have a roof over my head, legs that get me from A to B and a supportive family. I need to get some perspective . . . and also three pizzas and a tub of ice cream.'

Yes, the issues my clients were facing were far more urgent and serious than my waistline. They were also more important than me learning to speak to myself less horribly every day, and dragging around a tired, uncared-for body. But there is room for them both to matter. And, more importantly, they in fact have nothing to do with each other. Exercises like the ones you'll complete in this book showed me that I was always quick to find an 'out' by trivialising my relationship with food and my body because:

- Hearing disturbing stories all day was making me want immediate emotional relief from things like sugar to make me feel a bit better

- The fact I was already in a cycle of eating that left me craving unhealthy foods meant I was looking for any excuse to relieve myself from the sensation of physical withdrawal when trying to eat healthier ones

- I was looking for confirmation wherever I could find it that my body wasn't as worthy as everyone else's of being taken care of, and my problems were not as important

When you get to the section towards the end of this book which asks you to design and activate a practical plan of change, you will be starting something difficult, because it will be a change. You will face internal and external challenge. Even if every single meal you eat is delicious and healthy; even if you love completing the written exercises; even when you start to see results. There will still be moments when you tell yourself it's not as important to change as you thought it was that day when you swore you had to make changes once and for all.

At the end of this chapter, I am going to ask you to write a letter to yourself describing why things need to change. In this 'That's It' letter, you'll list as many reasons as you can think of why you want this to be last time you ever 'start again'. It'll be for your eyes only, so when it comes to completing it, be as honest as you can, and give importance to whatever you want. If, like me, you think that vanity will spur you on more than fear of heart disease, then that's absolutely fine. You're allowed to have whatever motivations you like, even if you're not proud of them. Plus, bear in mind, these won't be the same motivators that keep you going long term. Moving away from negative impacts just gets us going. It's the moving towards positive ones that keeps us going.

There's another reason why complete honesty and vulnerability with yourself is key here: we need a reliable baseline. I often mention how difficult it can be for even the most skilled, non-judgemental and compassionate therapists to create an environment in which people feel comfortable to tell the whole truth about the stuff they're not proud of straight away, without first building rapport. To give an honest and accurate picture of where they're starting from and how bad things can really get on the worst days. For obvious reasons (especially in my line of work that involved stigmatised and illegal activities), we often don't want to tell a complete stranger our true reasons for wanting to change or where our habits have taken us. But this also means that the therapist doesn't collect reliable information at the starting point, and therefore can't accurately measure our progress. Many smokers will be familiar with this. Clients have often told me that they've forgotten how much they downplayed the number of cigarettes they smoke per day to the GP during the last appointment. They forget their own lie. Then, even if they have cut down by the next appointment and report truthfully, their notes might say that they're smoking more than last time!

Moments of pride

Since you're doing this process on your own, you will be depriving yourself of a much-deserved pat on the back and celebration of milestones if you're not completely honest in this first exercise about things you're not happy with. For this process to work, you need to feel worthy. For that, you need to feel capable and strong.

To feel capable enough to face the challenges in this process and stay motivated, you'll need to be reflecting on and collecting examples of having felt proud of yourself. To feel authentically proud of yourself, you'll need to recognise when an accomplishment is truly an accomplishment for you personally. For that, you need to be completely honest about where you started.

When I look back on my own 'That's It' exercise, I still can't believe how many years I spent accepting and normalising all the tiny ways I was needlessly suffering every day. Seeing what I'd written at the start of this process reminded me that for most of my life, from the second I'd wake up in the morning, my weight was at the forefont of my thoughts. From how I felt as soon as I opened my eyes (anyone who is familiar with the late-night binge will tell you that this can cause a serious hangover), to what I said to myself when I looked in the mirror, to what clothes I chose to wear, to what assumptions I made about other people's responses and judgements towards me throughout the day, to my plan of whether to be 'good' or 'bad' with every single food choice. It was exhausting and constant and relentless.

While writing this book, I took a train journey that resulted in me going back and adding something I'd forgotten to add all those years ago to my 'That's It' letter:

So much of my brain space is taken up by how much physical space I'm taking up in lifts, on benches and cars.

I got on a tube line recently that I haven't taken for years, one where the seats don't have separators, and I saw one available next to the window. I simply walked through some people and over some bags, and sat down. This may sound ridiculous, but a few years ago, there's absolutely no way I would have done that. Even if my legs were aching and I had fifteen stops to take home. Why? Because this seemingly simple act of taking a seat would make me think this:

'All these other people will be looking at me scrambling around over them trying to get to that seat. They have nothing else to look at on this train so they'll be judging the hot and flustered giant fat woman wearing clothes that are too tight. The person I'd be sitting next to will be annoyed about all the space I'm taking up, plus my body will be pressed against theirs and they'll feel all my rolls. I won't be able to eat my sandwich because people will be thinking, "She shouldn't be eating that", and what if I have to get off the train before they do, which means I have to do that all over again?! Not worth it. I'll stand.'

I feel a mixture of sympathy for my former self and pride in my accomplishments when I notice that simple but grinding daily worries like whether to take a tube seat are things of the past. So, when highly personal realisations like this one come about, I go back to the exercise you'll do in this chapter and write down my observations. While I'm there, I glance at the other things too, just to help me remember to remember how far I've come. (And by the way, these days, even if for some reason I was three times the size I was at my heaviest, I would absolutely still push through everyone and take the tube seat with great joy. I know now that my lunch-needing, tax-paying, hard-working body deserves to sit down if it wants to – regardless of its size.)

The 'That's It' exercise in this chapter is the first of many to encourage you to think about how your relationship with your body and or eating habits is impacting various different areas of your life, and how these things might be inter-related. When people are completing this exercise, they commonly begin by thinking of the more obvious things they're not happy with, such as feeling unfit, uncomfortable or unattractive, or feeling out of control and emotionally, compulsively dependent on food. But I also ask that you consider the more subtle ones, such as the impact your diet has on your mental health and general sense of wellbeing, and what that means for your moods, and what your moods mean for your relationships with others, etc.

Applying this new kinder, more self-aware approach to weight management and body positivity involves getting really good at forward thinking. But I don't mean in terms of food choices. By forward thinking, I mean making decisions based on how we are likely to feel about them the next day, or week or month. To do this effectively, we need to understand how our habits impact each other. Sometimes we discover that habits we didn't even think were related to our eating patterns and body image are partly responsible for them.

Many of my clients realised after doing exercises like the one in this chapter that when choosing what to eat and drink in order to achieve the weight they want, they would have to limit their alcohol intake, not only for calorie reasons but also for resolve-lowering reasons. That's definitely something that was true for me – good luck getting me to look at a letter I wrote myself about why I want to lose weight when I'd had three glasses of wine and spotted a

McDonalds. Plus, drinking heavily made me wake up craving the kinds of foods that made me feel sluggish, anxious, bloated, disappointed – and wanting more.

By taking time to really capture how things are at their 'worst' for you in this exercise, you will create a powerful motivational tool to refer to when you feel challenged in the early stages of change, when the novelty of getting going may have worn off a bit. The letter you will write is to be written by past (and current you), for future you. While writing, try to visualise all times when you felt that you desperately want to change for good, when you've thought 'I never thought it would get to this stage. Something has to change once and for all.'

While I certainly don't want you to be feeling at your most fed up right at this second, it is those moments we want to capture for this exercise. For me, writing this letter involved thinking about crying in changing rooms, feeling too self-conscious and sweaty to dance at a wedding and walking home from the GP.

'That's It' Letter

I'd like you to now grab a notebook and write your own 'That's It' letter. Copy out and build on any of the following cues I've listed that makes sense for you personally. The more you write, the better. If you find yourself writing pages and pages, and going off on different branches from the first cue, go with it and see where it takes you! Don't feel under pressure to work through this or any of the other exercises in this book like a tick-box process or a questionnaire. They are designed to draw out wisdom you already have – not tell you exactly what to do.

They're here to help you be your own therapist and client at the same time. Let's go!

It's [insert date],

I've decided to try The Last Diet because . . .

I'm frustrated that . . .

Not making changes is negatively impacting my life in ways like . . .

Once and for all it's time to . . .

By now I thought I would have . . .

I know it would make me happier if I stopped . . .

Carrying on like this will mean that . . .

I would currently describe my relationship with food as . . .

I would currently describe my relationship with my body as . . .

I would currently describe my self-esteem as being . . .

At the moment my body feels . . .

Some of my reasons for wanting to change are things I don't want to share with anyone else. Things I'm not proud of. It's time to be honest with myself and admit that these include . . .

If, over the next weeks, I'm tempted to trivialise how important it is for me to change, I need to remember that . . .

I never thought I'd get to the stage where I'm . . .

If I start finding it harder than I expected, I want to remember it's important to push through because . . .

I need to take this seriously because . . .

There are other, related habits I'll need to change as well, these are things like . . .

I want to feel like I'm . . .

There are so many things that maintaining the status quo is holding me back from doing, like . . .

That's it!

[*Signature*]

Congratulations! You've started on your process of change! To mark the day you started The Last Diet, I suggest that you commit to introducing one tiny self-care ritual into your morning routine as of tomorrow. I mean tiny, and it needn't obviously have anything to do with losing weight. Anything that makes your body feel cared for and reminds you that things have changed as of today. It can be anything from setting a reminder alarm to stretch for one minute before you get in the shower, deciding to brew fresh coffee for yourself instead of grabbing the instant, or putting on music while you get ready for work. Something that reminds you that things have started to change for the better and you've embarked on a mission.

Ritual declaration

As of tomorrow I will _____ every day, just to make my life a little more pleasant. I'll remind myself to do it by _____.

no more mondays

Creating urgency to get going

I often hear people say, 'I know what I need to do, I just can't seem to get going.' I can absolutely relate to this. Especially when it comes to starting plans of change around eating habits and general self-care.

Until a few years ago, my life was essentially a cycle of full-bellied, well-intentioned, meticulously planned Sunday night resolutions, followed by deprived and emotional Mondays and finally compulsive, impulsive binges on foods I had deemed 'forbidden' by Tuesday night. That would continue on a loop until Sunday came around again. And of course, the Sundays kept coming around, and those binges added up over time to make me feel more weak, tired, out of control and disconnected from my body. The goals I set for myself were unrealistic, not suited to my body and didn't take into consideration that I'd wake up on Monday feeling hungry and lacking in emotional and physical resilience after another week of treating myself unkindly.

Often it took something as obvious as New Year's Eve or a birthday, or receiving an email from a boot camp I signed up to twenty-five Sunday nights ago to make me realise that with every week I said 'I'll start again on Monday', I was moving myself further away from having the relationship with my body that I ultimately wanted.

The mapping exercises later in this chapter are designed to help you bring about an urgency to change – that spark to 'get going'. They will involve you choosing a date in the future and mapping out two possible outcomes for yourself. Writing that date down will remind you that it's coming around whether you commit to making changes or not. First though, it is important to get excited about the future and remind yourself that this time around you're going to be considering how you can improve your wellbeing and prioritise self-care in every aspect of how you treat your body. That's what these next preparatory exercises will help you to do.

Written Exercise: No More Mondays: Part 1

For this first written exercise, answer the following question in as much detail as you can. Take time to paint a clear picture in your response, taking into consideration all the different life areas that you hope will have changed for the better:

In six months' time, if I asked the people closest to you what they've noticed has changed in terms of how you look and how you treat yourself, what would you like them to say?

_____

_____

_____

Let's now zoom in a little bit and start to get a clearer idea of your long-term goals in a nutshell, by using the following cues. Try to finish as many of these sentences as you can, depending on which are most relevant to you, and include as many different changes that come to mind.

Written Exercise: No More Mondays: Part 2

In six months' time, I want to be doing more . . .

_____

_____

_____

In six months' time, I want to be doing less . . .

_____

_____

_____

In six months' time, I want to be more . . .

_____

_____

_____

In six months' time, I want to be less . . .

_____

_____

_____

In six months' time, I want to feel more in control of . . .

_____

_____

_____

In six months' time, I want to have started . . .

_____

_____

_____

In six months' time, I want to have stopped . . .

_____

_____

_____

Briefly put, I'll know I've achieved my goals when I've:

_____

_____

_____

E.g. *changed my relationship with food, lost weight and started treating myself more kindly*

Map: No More Mondays: Part 3

Now, get out your notebook and in the middle of a blank page, write 'If I haven't . . .' followed by your final response in the part 2 exercise you just completed. Then write a date in the future underneath and draw a circle around them both together. When it comes to choosing what date to write, for the purpose of this exercise, I recommend six to twelve months from the date you wrote your 'That's It' letter.

If you're anything like me, this suggestion will immediately annoy you because it sounds like you won't be able to see results for ages. Worry not, when it comes to making practical changes to bring about any desired weight loss, you can go at whatever speed keeps you feeling strong and happy. Provided how you're eating helps your body to feel energetic, balanced and comfortable, you can design whatever eating habits are going to work for you and start losing weight immediately.

However, when it comes to addressing things that challenge the sustainability of your changes in the long term – like negative self-talk, self-sabotage and low self-esteem – there's no way around it: a deeper, more forward-thinking approach needs to be taken. One that considers all areas of your life and how you engage with the world around you as well as how you feel about your body. Irritating as it is, The Last Diet is the opposite of a crash diet, and there aren't any shortcuts. And while I'm already throwing around clichés about weight loss that used to annoy the hell out of me, I may as well share something I've observed in a lot of people trying to keep off lost weight: the quicker you lose it, the quicker you put it back on. Just my two cents.

Back to your map. Around the title and date you've already written, make notes to describe:

- How you are likely to be looking and feeling in your body if you haven't made changes

- The kinds of things you are likely to be saying to yourself and others about your body

- The kinds of things you are likely to be saying to yourself and others about how capable you are

- How your social life is likely to be looking

- How your relationships have been directly or indirectly impacted

- What the impact on your self-esteem is likely to be

- Ways you might have proven others – or yourself – right

- Ways your other habits may have changed as well

- Feedback you might be getting from those around you

- How you are likely to be spending your time, money and energy

- How you'll be feeling in general

When you're finished, put that map to one side for a moment.

Map: No More Mondays: Part 4

Now, on a new page, I'd like you to recreate the structure of the last map, writing down the same future date you chose before. The only difference is that you write 'If I have . . .' and again insert the same following sentence as before in the centre of the page, and draw a circle around it.

A note before you begin: try not to fall into the trap of simply populating this map with the opposite of what you wrote on the first map – in fact, put that map somewhere you can't see it. Think creatively about the many differences you might experience. Be ambitious for yourself; go into detail describing what this more favourable outcome would look and feel like for you across every possible life area. Describe:

- How you are likely to be looking and feeling in your body if you have made changes

- The kinds of things you are likely to be saying to yourself and others about your body

- The kinds of things you are likely to be saying to yourself and others about how capable you are

- How your social life is likely to be looking

- How your relationships have been directly or indirectly impacted

- What the impact on your self-esteem is likely to be

- Ways you might have proven others – or yourself – wrong

- Ways your other habits may have changed as well

- Feedback you might be getting from those around you

- How you're likely to be spending your time, money and energy

- How you'll be feeling in general

Reflection: No More Mondays: Part 5

Now, hold the last two maps side by side and compare the different outcomes. Note how it makes you feel to see the difference between them.

Although this exercise should bring about a sense of urgency to begin and stay on track, it will only be truly effective during this early part of the process, where I am assuming a few things may be the case:

- You're currently basing some or all of your worthiness to enjoy life on your body and/or your relationship with food

- You don't speak in a kind or encouraging manner towards yourself when you're not happy with how your body looks or how you've eaten

- You're highly alert to how other people may be judging your body or eating habits and still sensitive to what they think. Perhaps their voices or those of the media seem louder than yours, even when it comes to what choices you make for your body

- During times when you are neglecting or abusing your body in terms of food and exercise, you are taking an all-or-nothing and perhaps self-sabotaging approach to other areas of your life too

- You currently think that not looking how you want to look means you can't truly enjoy yourself in various settings

- You live life 'on hold' and still assume that there are certain things you can't do/wear/see/experience unless you've achieved weight-loss goals

From the next chapter onwards, the exercises I'm going to ask you to do will be focused on changing all of these beliefs about who you are, what you're capable of and what kind of life you deserve. That's why, soon, the comparison exercise you just did won't work quite as well again. Because by the end of this process you will have committed to disassociating your worthiness for joy, self-care and self-compassion from how you look or what you eat.

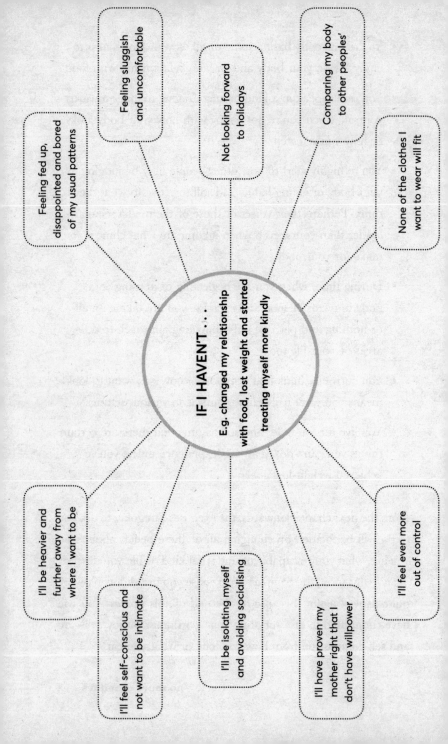

IF I HAVEN'T . . .
E.g. changed my relationship with food, lost weight and started treating myself more kindly

Feeling fed up, disappointed and bored of my usual patterns

Feeling sluggish and uncomfortable

Not looking forward to holidays

Comparing my body to other peoples'

None of the clothes I want to wear will fit

I'll be heavier and further away from where I want to be

I'll feel self-conscious and not want to be intimate

I'll be isolating myself and avoiding socialising

I'll have proven my mother right that I don't have willpower

I'll feel even more out of control

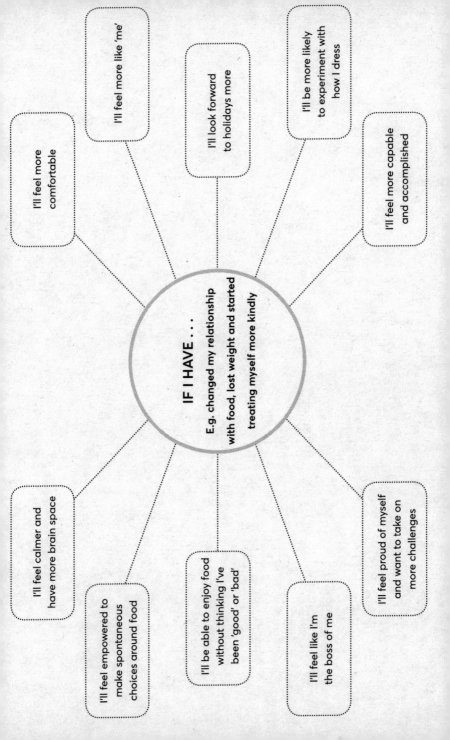

IF I HAVE . . .
E.g. changed my relationship with food, lost weight and started treating myself more kindly

I'll feel more comfortable

I'll feel more like 'me'

I'll look forward to holidays more

I'll be more likely to experiment with how I dress

I'll feel more capable and accomplished

I'll feel calmer and have more brain space

I'll feel empowered to make spontaneous choices around food

I'll be able to enjoy food without thinking I've been 'good' or 'bad'

I'll feel like I'm the boss of me

I'll feel proud of myself and want to take on more challenges

your body can

Losing weight is the least of what you're capable of

For many years, the only time I felt proud of my body was when it was managing to achieve a weight I was happy with, and look slim. I didn't acknowledge it in any other way – for example, when it managed to recover quickly after an operation. I didn't think the hair on its head deserved to be given care and attention unless it was growing out of the top of a slim face. If you asked me how much of my opinion of my body being attractive or healthy was tied up in my weight, for most of my life I would have said at least 90 per cent.

I've learned through my work that a lot of people can relate to feeling their opinion of their body is determined by their thoughts on what size they are. Most of us don't really stop to think about what our bodies have accomplished unless something is put in place to bring it to our attention. Perhaps giving birth or maybe a challenging physical expedition.

In the past, whenever I reached a goal weight, I'd feel temporarily euphoric. That day I would be on cloud nine. I wasn't at risk of succumbing to temptations. I felt strong because I was proud of myself and my body. Before long though, this would wear off and I wouldn't experience that powerful and euphoric feeling again until the next time the scales showed I'd lost weight.

I want to help you to change how you speak to your body about all it's capable of in addition to losing weight, so you can recreate that feeling of pride and therefore resilience every day. Think about the times when you talk to yourself and others about your body's abilities. How much of it is concerned with how it is serving you versus how it's not?

Naturally, this is partly because we take for granted our body's ability to complete basic functions. Many of us only come to acknowledge our bodies' power when it's brought to our attention how many people aren't as lucky. And when we go to the GP, it's remedial, it's to identify what's wrong, not what's strong. We're reminded every time we catch a common cold how debilitating and horrible it can be, yet when we're well we don't walk around saying, 'I'm really glad I don't have a cold today.'

This chapter is designed to help you realise that your body is more than capable of achieving your weight-loss goals, whatever they may be, and it provides an opportunity for you to record the amazing things your body has managed to accomplish in the past. Completing the 'My Body Can' map will mark the first step towards achieving the ultimate goal of shifting your thoughts so they focus on your assets more than your perceived deficits. It will remind you of how strong, resilient and useful your body is – and has always been.

Focusing on that evidence will help you to achieve your weight-loss goals far more effectively than focusing on what you wish your body didn't do, feel or look like. By shifting the focus from what you think your body can't do to what it can do, you will draw your attention to the unique combination of assets and resources you already possess. Some of which will play a direct role in you losing weight.

You will also learn to draw your attention more easily to all of your body's assets that are worthy of acknowledgment and care. Regardless of your size, your skin weathers tough conditions and deserves to be treated with care. Regardless of your weight, your spine deserves a stretching routine since it allows you to sit at a computer all day without having back problems. When you realise that your body has been your friend, and that all parts of it deserve to be treated well in every way, then what and how you eat becomes just one of those many ways.

One way to repay the favours your body has done (and to keep them coming) is to demonstrate more gratitude towards it across all areas of your life, and not just when it manages not to eat a second dessert or drag itself to the gym, but every day all day as it helps you navigate life.

Developing a kind attitude towards your whole body, one that takes the spotlight *off* your weight specifically, will actually help you to lose weight and keep it off. That's because the practice of identifying as many reasons as possible to treat all of your body well creates loads of opportunities to adopt a new range of kind habits. Ones that may not seem to have much to do with keeping off unwanted weight, but absolutely do. I believe that paying long-term attention to more subtle, seemingly unrelated self-care habits is what creates the stable foundation on which to maintain a weight you're happy with.

My process of successfully learning to care for my body regardless of its size has relied heavily on regularly bringing to my daily attention the ways in which I'm capable already. That's what the map in this chapter will help you to do for yourself. It's essentially a collection of ways your body has demonstrated that it's able to do difficult things.

Once you commit to regularly looking at and developing this map, you'll gradually notice a shift: what you're writing and reading about yourself will start to influence how you're thinking and feeling and behaving towards yourself. That's why, years from now, you'll only use this map as an ongoing record of your achievements and a motivational boost. You'll no longer need to refer to it immediately at times when your body feels challenged; you won't need regular visual reminders because you'll have developed a strong enough belief in your body to withstand short-term discomfort. You'll have developed a new habit of challenging your own self-doubting thoughts and beliefs by being able to quickly draw on recent and varied examples that disprove them. Examples of things your body has already achieved, survived and overcome. The times it's done you a favour without asking for much in return.

Map: My Body Can

I would like you to give this map a theme, by writing 'My Body Can' in the middle of a blank page, with a circle drawn around it. Then, note down your answers to the following questions anywhere you'd like on the page, drawing circles around each one of them as you go.

- What has your body managed to survive/endure/recover from over the years?

- What has your body helped/allowed you to accomplish?

- What has your body done to demonstrate how strong, resilient and capable it is?

- What does your body enable you to do on a daily basis?

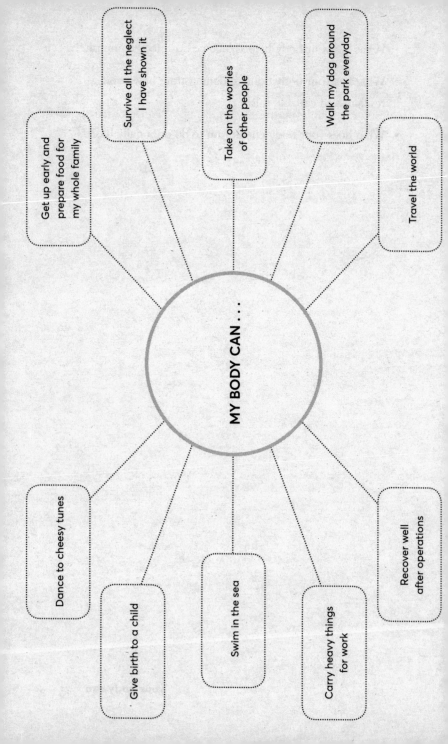

Written Exercise: My Body Deserves

Once you've acknowledged what your body is capable of, note down some suggestions of new self-care habits you could adopt to treat it with more gratitude. Ones that may not be directly related to diet or exercise. Anything from deciding to play music to please your ears while you do household chores to booking yourself a regular massage to thank your muscles.

1. _____

2. _____

3. _____

4. _____

5. _____

As with all of the exercises in this book, this one is intended to get the juices flowing. Ideally you will feel you are always on the search for new and practical ways to treat your body with the care and consideration it needs and deserves.

your body has

Focusing on your strengths

Now it's time to look at all the amazing things about your body; the purpose of this chapter is to apply this same principle to increasing your self-esteem by drawing your attention to the things you like about yourself. I will help you to create a collection of positive qualities that your body possesses. Learning to like yourself more will then help in convincing you that you're deserving of being treated with care, consideration and respect.

I often ask my clients to tell me how they think someone who really likes themselves and is happy in their body behaves on a daily basis. They often respond with suggestions like, 'They drink lots of water, they sit up straight, they take pride in their appearance, they're confident, they take vitamins, they are active and energetic, and eat things like vegetables and fish.'

This answer tells us two interesting things:

1. That whether or not they know how to keep it up, my
   clients already know what to do to practically lose weight.
   So even if they just *pretended* they were someone who liked
   themselves more, they'd probably manage to do that

2. That they believe being worthy of acting kindly towards their body in general is dependent on the weight and size of it at any given time. I know this because they automatically assume the person I'm asking them to describe in my question (the one who likes their body) is slim. I believe that in order to achieve long-term, sustained and meaningful weight loss, this belief needs to change

At some stage of our lives, for many different reasons, some of us started believing that being able to like our bodies was dependent on the size or weight of them. I won't patronise you by explaining why that's sad. But it's often why many people have a lot of unlearning to do when it comes to separating body weight and size from body likeability and worthiness. Years of ingrained habits will of course mean that there is often emotional and physical resistance and delay. For many of us, it is not as simple as adopting all the habits of a slim person. A deeper, more considered approach is needed to change how we think about our bodies.

But I don't want my clients and readers to have to wait until they've done loads of mindset shifting before they can get going with the actual weight loss. So I don't ask them to act like the person they *wish* they were. I simply ask them to immediately start realising and acting like the person they already are. I help them to do this by asking them to list all the things they like about all the different parts of their body, as you'll do later in this chapter.

One challenge faced by many clients who have learned to associate liking their bodies with being slim is that they struggle to identify positive qualities, especially at the times when they're not at a weight they want to be. They forget that their bodies are made up of eyebrows, skin, the shape of their forearms, their ankles, their toes, hair, muscles and other completely unique and beautiful features. Not to mention the qualities that have enabled them to accomplish the things they wrote on their 'My Body Can' map.

The idea is that when you look at a collection of positive qualities you already possess and things your body has managed to do, you can start to think, 'That is a person who deserves to be treated well. That is a person I imagine has a lot of self-esteem. That is a person who is totally capable and worthy of achieving any goal they like.' In this way, you can start to see the contrast between the person you actually already are, and the person you treat your body as though you are. When you focus on the qualities you don't possess, you're more likely to make the day-to-day choices of someone who doesn't feel worthy of aspiring to and achieving ambitious goals.

So this isn't just an 'it's nice to be nice' exercise. While you're busy creating tiny new habits that treat all of your body with the kindness it already deserves, you'll start to naturally enjoy the benefits you don't think it deserves (yet). Your body and mind can start taking care of the weight loss while you're busy taking care of your body and mind.

This idea of embodying who I already am was one of the earliest and most important shifts that helped me to lose weight both quickly and meaningfully. It came as a result of a therapy session I had when I was at one of my heaviest stages. I was once again telling the counsellor about all the things I intended to do when I was slim. Things like wearing nice jewellery and heels, going on dates, jogging in the park. And she asked me a question that really angered me: 'What if you're never slim?'

I can't tell you how much this suggestion enraged me. So much so that I drafted break-up messages during the days after this session. Not losing weight was simply not an option that had ever crossed my mind. For as long as I could remember, I believed that I could only truly enjoy my life when I was slim, and that during the stages when I wasn't slim, my main focus had to be getting slim again so I could enjoy my life again.

Once the anger subsided, I started realising that my way of thinking had resulted in me living huge chunks of my life completely 'on hold', not least since my slim phases were always very brief. By 'on hold', I don't even mean just not going out much because clothes didn't fit. I mean not lighting candles, not using nice face creams, not drinking nice bottles of wine, not listening to music. By assuming that these were only things people who liked themselves (because they were thin) did, I was depriving myself of so much self-care, enjoyment and motivation.

Many times when I was very overweight, I would buy clothes that were three sizes too small for me and hang them around my flat as a reminder of what I wanted to achieve. Any time spent not being slim was time spent planning to get slim again, without any consideration for the parts of my body that weren't directly related to losing weight.

So I made a list of the things I was waiting until I was slim to do, and really asked myself whether being able or worthy of doing them was dependent on my size. Turns out none of it was. I started doing the things on that list. It turned out that a lot of the habits I developed with the period of living life 'on hold' were actually contributing to my weight gain. Habits like being at home by myself for long periods either snacking mindlessly or starving while I browsed online for a dress I could maybe wear in four months' time if I stayed hungry until then.

Once I stopped living my life on hold, not only did I enjoy it more, but I lost weight more quickly than I had before. Embracing the kind habits I deserved, regardless of my size, across every possible aspect of my life actually made it difficult for the unkind food habits to fit in anymore. I noticed that when I lit those candles, put on that music, picked out that jumper I was keeping for a special 'thin' occasion or meditated for ten minutes, the environment wasn't so welcoming to unkind food habits. I discovered I could pepper my day with so much self-care that my stubborn unwanted eating habits – like eating compulsively out of anger or sadness – started looking and feeling out of place.

Here are some of the self-care habits that work for me at the time of writing this book. I change them every few months, as my routine and needs change or I discover something new I want to add.

When I wake up in the morning, I purposefully abstain from looking at my phone, and instead put out a yoga mat to have a stretch. I quite often consciously take a couple minutes more in the shower than I need to, just enjoy it. I try to make sure I eat some fruit, I moisturise my body well, use my favourite mug for coffee and take pride in my clothing choices – it then just doesn't feel right to eat three croissants mindlessly on the tube. It's like every time I make even the smallest kind choice for myself, it impacts the next one, and the one after that. It just so happens that over the course of every day, some of my choices involve food and exercise. They're just mixed in with all the kindness.

There's less resistance to change when you've made it easy to slot new eating habits into an established self-care framework. The following exercise will help you feel more deserving and motivated to create that framework.

Map: My Body Has

First I'd like you to write 'My Body Has' in the middle of the page with a circle drawn around it. Then simply start noting down all the things you like about any and every aspect of your body, drawing circles around each one of those as you go. What bits of it do you like and why? Which would you not like to change and why? Try to keep your entries as brief as possible on this map. No more than a few words for each one.

Note: When you start writing these down, notice any caveats that pop up. Do you feel resistance when you try to believe you really possess positive qualities? Perhaps you went to write 'beautiful hair' and immediately thought, 'Well it could be better, it does need a cut, it's never been as shiny as my sister's.' All I ask for now is that you notice that, and write down the positive quality nonetheless.

Learning to own and believe in our positive qualities is a hugely important part of this process. Firstly of course because we deserve to focus on what we like about ourselves and it makes for a nicer life. But also because when we feel totally secure in the knowledge that we possess loads of indisputably positive qualities, we can take on useful advice and criticism more easily without becoming defensive. In my experience, the people who are most willing to consider how they could change for the better are the ones who feel very clear in why they like themselves whether or not they change.

When you've completed this map you'll have a collection of your body's self-identified positive qualities. The idea is that glancing at this will help you want to create more self-care habits – at moments when you want to neglect or do a disservice to your body's needs in any way, I want you to look at it and think, 'That's a body worth treating well.'

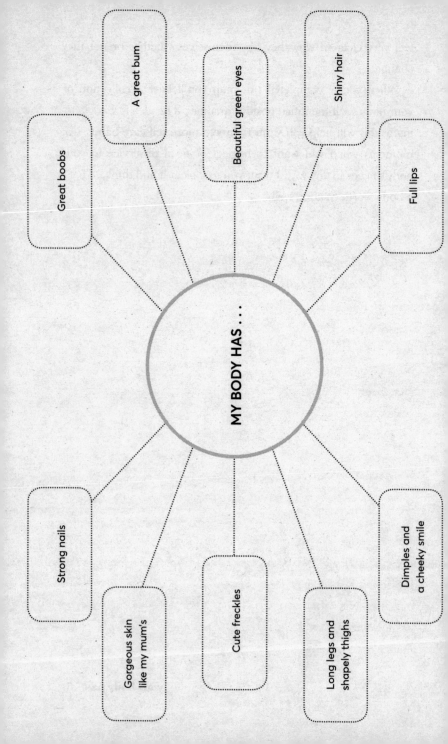

your soundtrack

Turning urges from commands into alerts

People often come to me because their behaviour around food and abuse of their bodies has made them feel out of control. They feel they are trapped in a cycle of behaving in ways they don't want to and that they can't withstand the short-term physical and emotional discomfort of making changes for long enough to see meaningful and lasting results. Clients often describe their urgent, compulsive and impulsive actions towards their bodies when it comes to eating habits as being very reactionary: when the physical craving or emotional need arises they feel powerless.

A big part of adopting The Last Diet effectively is realising that our actions are determined by internal commands and conversations that we have with ourselves. Ultimately, we decide whether to act in a certain way. It doesn't matter how hungry we are and how delicious something we're trying to avoid looks, that craving doesn't physically force our hands to pick it up and eat it. What happens is, we tell ourselves a story about the situation, and about ourselves. This often happens very quickly, and so it isn't until we acknowledge that it is happening, look at our patterns and externalise what's going on that we can start to slow down the decision-making process when it comes to how we act towards our bodies. We can commit to turning a physical or emotional craving into an alert as opposed to a command. We do this by compassionately and curiously examining what those commands are and where they came from, before practising ways to catch them, change them and create new ones.

When I began to look consciously at my internal commands, I found the shift that it brought about to be life changing. By doing exercises like the ones in this book to change the conversations I have with my body, I have changed how I speak to myself about everything. That's the thing with The Last Diet; as soon as you really commit to practising the self-awareness and self-esteem tools, you find yourself using them in every other possible area of your life.

Through working with clients to change their habits around food, I have come to realise that we all have a very unique internal soundtrack playing most of the time. One that's made up of assumptions and beliefs about ourselves, others and the situations we're in. One that ultimately dictates how we act. When we're faced with the decision of how to react to a challenging situation or feeling, that soundtrack becomes very important.

Despite how long we've spent beating ourselves up for it, I have been very pleasantly surprised at how quickly myself, and my clients who want to lose weight, have been able to change years of negative self-talk. I think that may be because, when working with issues of weight, we have so many opportunities to practise throughout the day! Being challenged with constant food choices turns up the volume on our soundtrack; it helps us to listen in on our commands more clearly and notice the same unhelpful ones popping up over and over again. If you have spent a lifetime listening to a negative soundtrack about your body and eating habits, you'll have many opportunities throughout the day to listen in on what it is telling you to do.

Applying The Last Diet to change your commands about food will of course help you to lose as much weight as you'd like. To keep it off however, you need to feel capable. For that to feel authentic, you need evidence of having survived physical cravings and self-doubt and come out the other side unharmed. Since short-term discomfort is a volume-increaser on our internal commands, one way to gather new evidence of how resilient you are in general is this:

1. Pick a habit you want to change

2. Identify the challenges you're most sceptical about being able to overcome when trying to change

3. Decide that you'll now be consciously facing these challenges head on, and putting yourself in that discomfort on purpose. Not for something as basic as losing weight, but so that you can do a check-in on the current unhelpful commands you have about them

Challenges turn up the volume and give us invaluable insight into why we're finding it so difficult to change. We just have to choose to tune in on purpose and with purpose. The smallest tweaks to the status quo can be used to turn up those conversations you have with yourself and draw out the wisdom you need to change your commands.

One of my clients recently described how she noticed her internal dialogue change as a result of applying just two of my suggestions to her daily routine: 1) First thing in the morning, look in the mirror and acknowledge one thing you like about your body out loud. 2) When 4pm comes around, have three fingers of KitKat instead of all four as you usually would.

I received an email from this client one week after our first session, reporting her findings:

Hi Shahroo,

So, I tried out the mirror and KitKat missions. To be honest, when I left our session I thought they sounded too easy. Then I tried them and was shocked to discover what I did.

When I tried to stand in front of the mirror and say out loud just one thing I liked about my body, I heard:

This is so stupid.

Who are you kidding? This self-love stuff isn't for you. Just stop eating so much.

This is actually making me notice more things I don't like about myself.

Eurgh, I feel gross, I don't want to do this.

I'm just going to say whatever. My eyebrows. Although my aunt always used to say they were an odd shape.

You already look awful, who cares what you put in your body.

When I tried to leave one finger of KitKat in the afternoon, I heard:

You're not the kind of person who can just leave it. You never have been.

People are starving in the world, just eat it.

This is stupid, you can start tomorrow.

You need it, you're stressed.

You should eat it, you're already being bad for eating KitKats at all.

As you can see, the commands I'm giving myself don't have my best interests at heart. They don't have much faith in me at all.

For this client, it was incredibly impactful to realise that her internal dialogue was making the process of change so much more difficult than it needed to be. After the initial shock of how unhelpful she'd been to herself in her soundtrack, she resolved to create tiny tweaks across various areas of her life, just to turn up the volume and check in with what she'd been telling herself she could do or could not do without even realising.

How you speak to yourself in general will determine whether you get back on track – and stay there – in the event that you deviate from your weight-loss plan. Let's say for example you've stuck to an eating plan that you're really happy with. You've been following your own guidelines for two weeks – so long enough to feel proud of yourself, but not long enough to have addressed and changed all-or-nothing thinking patterns and self-sabotaging messages about food and your relationship with it. You get invited to a dinner party at someone's house and when you get there, you realise that eating anything they've cooked would mean you went off-plan. You don't say anything, and decide you have no choice but to eat it. You know, logically, rationally speaking, that this one evening will not derail all of your efforts to date. You know that one meal will not be responsible for weight gain. What *will* be responsible for it is what you do after that meal. The twenty meals you choose to have after it will depend on the conversation you have with yourself; what you tell yourself that one meal meant about you and the situation you were in.

There will come a point in this process when you will need to identify more practically, clearly and in detail what eating plan you would like to implement in order to lose weight. As you will have gathered by now, I believe it's no business of mine what you decide to eat or not eat and how many times (if any) you decide to exercise in order to reach your goals. My focus will be on helping you to identify which of these three conditions you are in in relation to your chosen 'way of eating' at any given time:

1. On track

2. Lapse

3. Relapse

Later on, you will have more clarity on what each of these conditions looks like for you. Broadly speaking, being 'on track' means that you're keeping to whatever eating, exercise and personal development plan you've assigned for yourself. Lapsing is a deviation from this plan and relapsing is when you've fully returned to old, unwanted habits.

The conversation we have with ourselves determines whether a lapse turns into a relapse. In this process, mastering lapse management by changing your internal commands will enable you to master weight management and still enjoy the more fattening foods you love. I now manage my weight practically speaking, by spending about 70 per cent of the time sticking to whatever my 'on track' is and 30 per cent lapsing at will, safe in the knowledge I'll immediately get back on track.

Since my internal dialogue no longer tells me to lapse again immediately (and even if it does, I've demonstrated it's not the boss of me), my weight isn't affected. By using the exercises in this book, I've learned to 'listen in' on my commands and self-doubting thoughts, and challenge them with genuine facts; I've developed a bullshit filter for all-or-nothing, self-sabotaging thinking. I still hear it now and then, but it just doesn't put forward a compelling argument. Just because I had one meal and woke up predictably craving sugar doesn't mean I am forced to not get back on track immediately.

In the next exercise, you shine a light on how you've been speaking to yourself in those moments when the script is most important. This will in turn help you understand the kinds of commands you'll be giving yourself about what the next step should be after a lapse. Resist the temptation to downplay any parts of your internal conversation because it causes you discomfort when you see it all written down. One of the unfortunate realities of making meaningful shifts by becoming more self-aware is that sometimes things have to get a tiny bit harder before they get a whole lot easier.

Map: My Soundtrack: Part 1

Start by writing 'My Soundtrack' in the middle of a blank page with a circle around it. Now, think back to times when you've attempted to change your eating and exercise habits but failed to keep it up. What kinds of things did you say to yourself in those moments when you realised you'd 'failed' at keeping up your plan? Write down the messages you give yourself in those moments and draw a circle around each one as you go.

Next, move on to the things you say to yourself in general when you're finding something more difficult than you think you should, or you feel you've let yourself down in some way. For example, if you make a mistake at work, or snap at a loved one and later feel guilty about it.

Finally, write down the things you say about your body specifically when you don't manage to stick to a weight-loss or exercise plan.

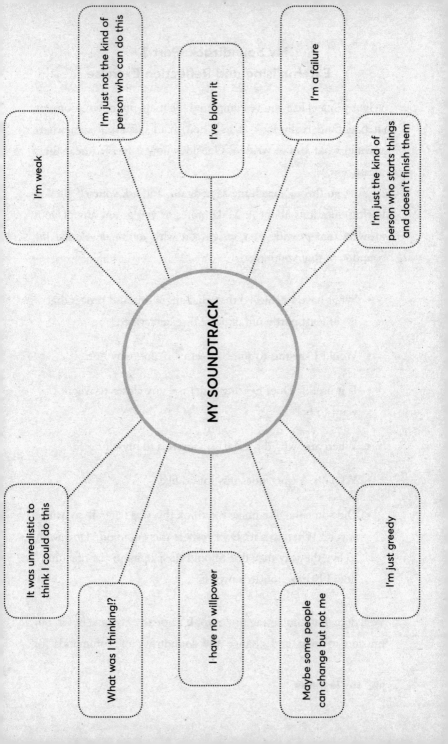

MY SOUNDTRACK

I'm weak

I'm just not the kind of person who can do this

I've blown it

I'm a failure

I'm just the kind of person who starts things and doesn't finish them

It was unrealistic to think I could do this

What was I thinking!?

I have no willpower

Maybe some people can change but not me

I'm just greedy

My Soundtrack: Part 2 –
Externalising and Reflection Exercise

When you feel like you've completed the map, put down your pen, sit back and really look at it. Then, read out loud (somewhere private) what you've written. Consider how it feels to hear these messages.

Now, go through each message again, and ask yourself the following questions about it. Make notes as you go on any of your answers that provide new insight on why you've developed the soundtrack that you have.

- What have I achieved that challenges this and proves that it's at least partly unfair, false or exaggerated?

- Would I say this to someone else? If not, why not?

- Is it useful? Does hearing it get me any closer to where I want to be?

- When and why did I start saying this to myself?

- Who else's voice does this sound like?

- Did someone else make me think this was true? If so, who was it? When was it? Do I respect their opinion? Do I want to live the way they do? Should their opinions be dictating how I behave towards myself?

Well done for completing this map. It's not an easy one, but in our mission to hear and change the soundtrack of commands for good, we've got to first understand what we're up against – and that's often years of outdated, unhelpful, untrue yet truly compelling core beliefs about ourselves and what we're capable of. Finishing this chapter is a good opportunity to acknowledge that you no longer want to speak to yourself unkindly. That you realise now it's unhelpful in every possible way. That you will commit to observing then questioning any cruel or unfair assumptions about how capable you are of achieving even your most ambitious weight-loss goals. And that you will reframe tiny challenges throughout your day as opportunities to choose to check in with how you're speaking to yourself.

cheerleading

Becoming your own motivational coach

When it comes to supporting the people we care about, most of us think we know how to give decent advice and that we recognise what kinds of messages make people feel strong, empowered, resilient and able to overcome a hurdle. But for various reasons some of us developed a habit of not applying that same wisdom when it came to supporting ourselves. We became skilled at being able to sit in front of our loved ones and tell them that they are capable and strong and worthy of achieving ambitious goals, all the while showing ourselves in how we behave towards our own bodies that we don't think we are capable or strong or worthy of doing the same.

I often ask my clients how they would react if someone they loved and respected was beating themselves up about having behaved in a way they weren't happy with. Without fail, everyone responds that they would say things like 'Don't worry about it! You didn't set out to do it! These things happen, don't beat yourself up about it! Worrying won't change anything, everyone makes mistakes, this doesn't deserve to ruin your day.' And yet very few people can recall the last time they spoke to themselves like this when they had a blip and lapsed from a healthy eating plan, forgot someone's birthday or made a blunder at work.

Making changes is hard, especially in the early stages. Your motivation to stay on track will waver and you will need pep talks. You'll need reminders of why you're doing this and why it's important, as well as why you're capable of withstanding short-term discomfort to achieve your long-term goals. Essentially, you'll need a wise, protective, enthusiastic coach who has every faith in you and keeps you motivated around the clock. Since you're the only person who's with you twenty-four hours a day (plus you're the only one who truly knows all of your most private of motivations) you're the best candidate for the job.

Before you can start though, you'll need a script. Because you may well have discovered in the last chapter that your current script won't motivate anyone to do anything for long. You'll also need to hand yourself over to the process a little bit, and push through the initial discomfort of how unnatural it feels to encourage and motivate yourself. You may well find it difficult to feel that you deserve to be supported and championed in the same way that someone you love deserves to be supported and championed. So, to get around that possible stumbling block, we're now going to draw that motivating script out of you – the one you already know.

Map: Cheerleading: Part 1

First, think of someone you love dearly. Someone you really believe in and for whom you wish nothing but success. A person you would be prepared to help in any way they needed if it meant they could be happier. Write their name down in the centre of a blank page in your notebook and draw a circle around it.

Then, imagine this person comes to you and says that they're struggling to lose weight and it's really upsetting them. They don't think they're capable of achieving their goals and don't feel like they deserve success. They tell you that they don't have the strength to stay on track and feel disappointed in themselves for lapsing so often. Imagine your task is to help them get back on track and believe in themselves as quickly as possible. Write down everything you would say to them, and what you'd advise them to do. Draw a circle around each statement as you go along.

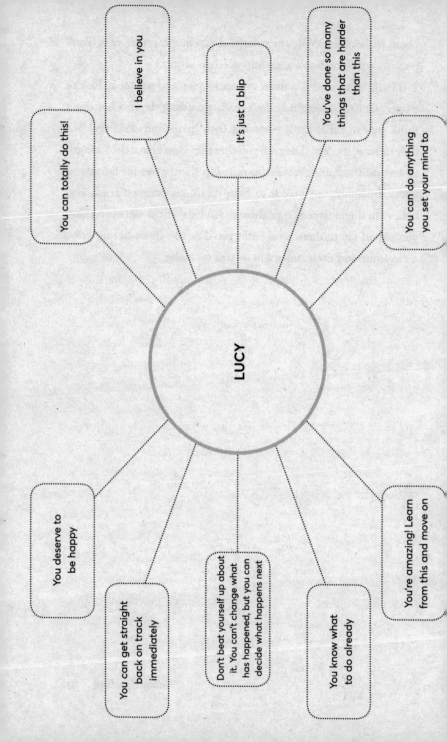

Reflection: Cheerleading: Part 2

When you've finished your 'Cheerleading' map, get out your 'My Soundtrack' map and compare the two. The Cheerleading map shows the messages you believe motivate people and the My Soundtrack map shows the messages you give yourself in the moments when you need motivating. So now you can start asking yourself the question, why do your loved ones deserve motivational messages of encouragement that get them back on track quickly, and you don't?

Throughout this process, you will be faced with challenging moments when you want to throw in the towel, delay starting or believe the self-doubting messages you give yourself. It's in those moments that it's most important that you step into that role of motivational coach. Where you decide you're going to be your own best friend and choose new messages and commands to give a body that you are learning to love and respect more every day. The good news is you already know how to motivate someone you love. You have the script there on your Cheerleading map.

For many people, reflecting on these two exercises brings to their attention that their inability to achieve their weight-loss goals was never about being unable to motivate themselves. It was about not caring enough about their bodies to feel worthy of hearing the messages they needed to hear in order to get through the tough times. It was about unconsciously obeying all-or-nothing, self-defeating commands and framing a lapse as a failure as opposed to something that can be learned from, engaged in consciously and, most importantly, immediately bounced back to 'on track' from.

I have found time and time again that the simplest way to start helping people treat and speak to themselves with more kindness all day and in every way is to pretend they are living in the body of someone they love.

One of my clients was a single father who worked long hours and found it difficult to manage the stress of day-to-day life without taking comfort in convenient fast food, even though he felt it was making him feel sluggish and irritable with his children and his colleagues. His food choices were causing him to gain unwanted weight. He would snack throughout the day on the same stuff; mainly foods that gave him a quick hit but then caused his energy levels to slump. He would eat mindlessly and on the go, not taking time to present his meals in a way that made them look appealing. He wanted to lose weight in order to feel more mobile when playing with his children and to set a good example for them, so he came to me for help.

I noticed during our first conversation that many of his reasons to change involved giving his children the best possible quality of life. He knew that taking better care of his body was the way to be able to do that long term, but when it came to his day-to-day choices for himself, his own needs were always last when it came to the smallest acts of kindness, respect and consideration.

So I set him this mission: imagine one of your daughters is living on her own for the first time. She's setting a precedent and creating a new 'normal' for how she will treat her body and what kind of routine she will have when no one is there to supervise her anymore. This includes how often she exercises or gets some fresh air; what choices she makes when she wants a snack; how she consumes alcohol and sugar; how much time and consideration she takes choosing ingredients for the meals she makes. Imagine her sitting down eating a meal at dinnertime. How would you like to think her food would be presented, and how would she be eating it? Would it be in a rushed manner, grabbing whatever she can get that gives her a quick fix? Or in a mindful way where she can show her body respect?

Once he had imagined it in detail, I asked the client to simply resolve to spend the next week treating himself as he'd like his daughter to treat herself when it came to food, exercise and general wellbeing decisions. I asked that whenever he went to buy an unhealthy snack, he considered whether he'd want his daughter to make that same choice for her body. I asked that when it came to deciding whether to put in the extra time and effort to prepare a meal from scratch for himself (one that he knew would be better for his body and mind than one that took two minutes to make), he made the same decision he'd want his daughter to make for herself.

After three weeks or so, I heard back from this client and he told me he was still doing the exercise every day. He said that it helped him open his eyes to all the healthier substitutes there were available when he wanted a snack – he had just needed to give it a bit more thought. And he hadn't realised quite how little he cared for his body until he saw how many times a day he was treating it extremely differently to how he'd want someone he loved to treat theirs. Naturally he'd also lost weight, but as is the case with all of my clients, achieving the goals they initially set out to achieve quickly becomes a bonus, a by-product of learning to treat themselves more kindly in every possible way throughout the day.

not your bag

Acknowledging the approaches
that don't work for you

I don't know about you, but I feel extremely overwhelmed with how much conflicting advice is going around when it comes to the healthiest way to lose and manage weight. The majority of clients who come to me for help with weight loss are like me in that they've spent many years trying out different methods. They're always keen to hear about a new miracle diet or exercise programme. All of my clients, regardless of whatever has proven successful in helping them to lose weight in the past, share one thing in common: they haven't yet found a 'normal', 'healthy' way of eating long term that enables them to maintain weight loss while also enjoying the more fattening foods that they love.

Whenever I ask clients why they think past plans failed to keep them at a weight they were happy with, they describe different elements of each plan that simply weren't realistic, sustainable or appealing. In other words, keeping up their new 'healthier' habits involved continuing to hand themselves over to a prescriptive plan, some elements of which they could get on board with long term and others that they couldn't. But they never stopped to consider whether they could pick and choose the parts of these plans that they liked, not based on what they were told about them, but based on how they had responded to them time and time again.

There have been so many occasions throughout my life when I've sat at a laptop, or at a notebook with different coloured pens, planning meticulously how I'd wake up at 7am, go for a run, then make a fresh grapefruit juice (because I read when I was twelve that it burns fat). How I'll then have a warm glass of water with lemon followed by whichever breakfast made with nine different expensive ingredients (seven of which I don't even like) is required by the diet I'm following right now.

I've since learned that when attempting to design the most painless and enjoyable weight-loss plan possible for ourselves, the answers lie in the wisdom we've developed from past experience. Some plans will have made us feel bored after a while, others may have left us lethargic, or often feeling like we had to isolate ourselves and avoid socialising to keep it up.

This next exercise is the one I did right before I created the eating and exercise plan that finally helped me lose weight once and for all. First I made a list of all the diets I'd tried in the past, and then, next to each one, I wrote down why I thought I didn't manage to keep it up.

I decided that, for once, instead of thinking there was something wrong with me and presuming I'd one day transform into someone else, I would be honest with myself about who I was today. And who I have demonstrated myself to be when it comes to trying to change my relationship with food and my body in the past. I entertained the possibility that maybe I didn't need to change to accommodate the plan, but that the plan needed to change to accommodate me.

This is the list I initially made of the kinds of plans that hadn't worked for me in the past, with some of my reasons why. I simply based these reasons on who I was at the time of starting, and how I'd always shown myself to behave and react prior to that.

Things that I discovered weren't my bag:

- Eating plans that suggested I cut out a lot of the foods that I loved forever if I wanted to maintain my weight loss

- Having to measure and weigh my food

- Anything that stopped me going out to eat at restaurants

- Plans that didn't involve eating solid food

- Diets that required me to purchase specific bars and sachets and supplements

- Exercise classes that required me to wake up early in the morning

- Meal plans that required me to cook complicated things

- Plans that didn't let me drink coffee

- Plans that didn't let me drink alcohol

- Diet plans that technically allowed me to consume huge amounts of things that you don't have to be a nutritionist to know isn't right (I've been known to snack on canisters of whipped cream because it's permitted)

- Diets that focus so much on not combining certain foods that I'm made to feel one wrong decision will ruin the whole thing (I didn't need to be adopting approaches that reinforce my all-or-nothing thinking)

- Plans that permitted me to still eat my usual binge foods daily and expected me to miraculously be able to eat them in more moderate quantities

- Plans that said I had to stop eating many hours before I go to bed (going to bed hungry bothers me so much that it has genuinely been known to make me emotional)

- Having to measure myself with a measuring tape (I'd always lose them, plus I have the kind of body that can sometimes look seven months pregnant for a few hours after even an undisputedly healthy meal. Wrongly timed measuring could be demoralising)

- Having to eat the same thing over and over again (I still can't really be around cabbage soup without feeling sick)

- Having to report to someone for a public weigh-in (this reinforced my inclination to want to binge straight after being weighed, safe in the knowledge I wouldn't be monitored again for another six days)

I can't stress enough that I haven't shared this list in the hope you will use the same ones. I simply want to show you an example of how a plan of eating can be designed from a place of honest self-acceptance, with your bespoke needs in mind. Losing weight and finding a routine that keeps it off is difficult enough, the last thing you need is for your plan to include things that experience has regularly shown don't work for you.

It's also important to note that I wrote this list very early on, when I had not yet developed an ability to challenge all-or-nothing thinking, or the tools to motivate myself to go out to exercise even if it's cold. I also didn't appreciate the value of waking up earlier. These are things I feel much more able to do now, but I'm still so glad that, back when I made the list, I gave myself the best possible chance at getting through the difficult initial stages of change by facing up to the things that don't work for me, and accepting myself just as I was.

Recently, I had a consultation with a new client. She came in (as most clients do) feeling very clear on what her goals were. She wanted to lose three stone as quickly as possible so she could feel her best for her upcoming fortieth birthday party. She said, 'I read that you help people who already know what they want to do and how they want to do it. So, all I need from you is to help me understand why I can't keep up this eating and exercise plan. I always get to day thirteen and give up. I need you to help me understand how to be less weak so I can do this.'

I looked at the plan she had written down in her notebook. It included eating different meals to the ones she prepared for the rest of her family, missing breakfast despite having extremely busy mornings that required her to be focused at work, snacks that sounded as appealing as cardboard and so on. I asked her where she had got this plan from and she replied that it had always been her go-to plan to shed a few pounds since she was fifteen years old. Not only had the landscape of her life changed since then, but the needs of her body had too. She was beating herself up for not being able to keep up a regime that was already challenging when she had no bills to pay, no children to care for and very little to make her want to throw in the towel other than hunger on a day-to-day basis.

So I asked her why she kept going back to the same plan despite having totally different needs (and it clearly not working in a sustainable way to begin with). Her response: 'I was weaker then, it wasn't the right time to change, I didn't want it badly enough. Now I feel like I can really focus on this because I want to lose weight so badly.'

Instead of thinking there was something wrong with the plan, she thought there was something wrong with her. Plus, she assumed that increased desire, desperation and urgency were enough to keep her on track this time, despite it never working before. I invited her to start again. To consider that her weight-loss plan choices could be the ones that create the path of least resistance and make the journey less difficult.

I asked her when she needed to be more energetic, when she felt at her most resilient against temptation in the day, what foods she absolutely didn't want to cut out so she could enjoy her life and not fixate on them, how her body and tastes had changed over the years. What we created together was a plan that not only looked much kinder than her outdated, restrictive one based on generic guidelines, but that also helped her lose weight more effortlessly than she had ever imagined. It was bespoke and it worked for her – not the other way around.

The 'Not My Bag' list that you will now create in map form should take into consideration your inclinations and unique set of life circumstances – even if this includes things about yourself and your life that you ultimately want to change as well. For now, just accept the current situation so you can get going with a plan of action that yields results as soon as possible. Perhaps you have children, and so diets that require you to prepare separate meals aren't your bag. Maybe the industry you work in will always require you to attend a lot of late dinners, so a plan that demands you always know what is in your food and how it has been prepared might not be your bag – at least for as long as you have that job.

The exercise you complete now will invite you to reflect on previous attempts to lose weight or make changes to your relationship with food and your body. Think about what hasn't worked in the past and honestly ask yourself what things you simply don't want featuring in the eating, exercising and personal development plan you are going to design to help you lose and keep off weight.

Map: Not My Bag

First, write 'Not My Bag' in the centre of a blank page and draw a circle around it. Then think back to previous attempts and write why you don't think they worked for you long term.

To get the juices flowing and jog your memory, you may find it useful to ask yourself these questions:

- What elements of it weren't suited to my lifestyle?

- What was unrealistic about it?

- What aspects of it didn't suit my body?

- What aspects of it didn't suit my personality?

- What circumstances or events led up to me going off track eventually?

- How come I didn't get back on track when things started going wrong?

When you've taken time to note down all the things that aren't your bag, you will have a collection of personal wisdom that you can apply when it comes to formulating the best weight-loss and maintenance plan for you specifically. When creating your plan of least resistance, you'll already know what elements just aren't going to work for you, so you either rule them out or find an alternative. You'll create the plan it's most difficult to rebel against, since it's truly bespoke and based on self-knowledge and internal wisdom.

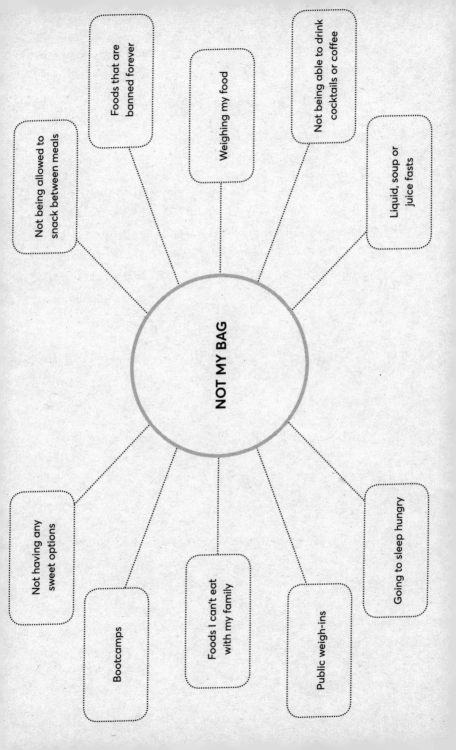

your style

Creating a plan of least resistance

Now that we've considered what doesn't work for you when it comes to losing and keeping off weight, we're going to look at what does. We'll do this by thinking about what kinds of plans tend to get you excited and make you want to keep them up across all areas of your life. The unique combination of circumstances to give you the best chance of achieving your weight-loss and maintenance goals.

Some people find it useful to declare their plans to others as this keeps them feeling accountable. Others find that this creates an added pressure and deprives them of the empowering feeling of being on something of a secret mission. When it comes to food, some people like to graze all day; others know it's best for them to eat three proper meals. Some people find that ramping up the exercise at the beginning of a new eating plan is an effective added motivator; others want to stay away from Lycra, mirrors and feeling out of breath until they've got past the initial adjustment stages of changing how they eat.

In this chapter you will start to think about what you'd like 'your style' to be when it comes to how you change and maintain your weight. The 'My Style' exercise you complete will not simply be a case of noting down the opposite of what you wrote on your 'Not My Bag' map. It will go further by asking you to consider the conditions you have shown yourself to thrive in across all areas of your life in the past. It will invite you to reflect on all of your proudest accomplishments to date – particularly the things that required you to push through (some of which you will have written on your 'My Body Can' map) – and think about what supports and resources you had in place at the time, both internally and externally.

What was it that made you stay on track in those moments when you wanted to give up? Did you have a deadline to work towards? Or someone else you were doing it for? Was it that you were organised and spent time planning properly, or perhaps that you were checking in with some kind of support network? How did you feel in yourself; did you have a self-care routine? Did you have any routine at all? Or do you feel at your most productive and motivated when free to make more spontaneous decisions? Did your most productive times happen to occur when something in particular was going on in a seemingly unrelated area of your life? Perhaps when you think back to your most productive and motivated periods they were during times when you were also taking more pride in your appearance and your surroundings.

I certainly find that the times when I'm feeling most resilient generally coincide with periods when my home environment is organised and aesthetically pleasing to me. I know that my enjoyment of seeing flowers in my flat first thing in the morning plays an indirect role in helping me to make kind decisions in my food choices later that day. How much time I take to brew my coffee so it's really delicious and do my hair so I like how it looks also play a role in the decisions I make regarding my eating habits and how I speak to my body once I've left the house. That's because these tiny acts of self-care are signals reminding me that I am worthy of taking care of in every way. That my quality of life matters. That my body is worthy of feeling its best, and therefore also eating in ways that makes it feel strong, happy, energetic and calm.

In taking time to consider what you'd like 'your style' to be when it comes to eating and exercise, you are also giving yourself an opportunity to consider what activities and conditions make you feel positive and resilient in general, so you can bring about the ones that are in your control and strive to create as many new ones as possible. When it comes to maintaining the resilience we need to change ingrained habits around food and resist temptation, especially during the early stages of change, trying to feel good in every possible way is an incredibly effective motivational tool for staying on track.

I can't help but notice that when it comes to weight-loss plans, almost all of my clients find it absurd if I suggest they start on Sunday as opposed to Monday. I understand, since I used to be like this too. It makes sense, because usually Monday is when our routines start up again and when we are less likely to feel idle and prone to mindless eating. Plus we associate the weekends with comfort and lack of restrictions, so why would we embark on the first day of a difficult plan when we're meant to be doing whatever we like?

The thing is, we know that we're better at doing difficult things when we're feeling strong, positive and energetic. Now, some people will feel this way on a Monday morning, and so it would make sense to embark on day one of a challenging eating plan then. For many people, however, Monday morning is associated with feeling sluggish, accompanied by a desire to ease back into the working week as gently as possible. So now I don't ask clients what day or time they'd like to start their plan. I simply ask them to tell me the day when they think they'll feel most positive, energetic and resilient. Their response is what I use to assign their day one.

Throughout this process, difficult choices will present themselves, often out of nowhere. The best you can do to prepare for them is to believe in your ability to overcome unforeseen challenges while doing what you can to create a practical plan of least resistance for you personally. The next exercise will help you to do that.

Map: My Style

First, write 'My Style' in the centre of a blank page, with a circle drawn around it. Then start to write down answers to these questions and cues, drawing circles around each response as you go:

- Think back to the periods when you've stuck to a difficult task in order to achieve a long-term goal. Write down the factors that you feel kept you on track

- Think back to the times you've been 'in the zone' with a weight-loss plan. Write a description of how things looked for you, internally and externally, that meant you could succeed, at least for a while

- Consider if there are any types of exercise you've not minded sticking to for a while in the past, and why you think that was

- Write down some delicious meals that you consider healthy. Ones you believe you can enjoy eating while still losing weight

- Write down your personal tastes when it comes to food choices. Is it important for you to eat something sweet after dinner? Are you someone who wants a diet that is heavy in meat?

- Think back to a time in your life when you've felt really capable for an extended period of time. Note down what it was about the activity that made you feel accomplished and proud of yourself

Once you've completed this exercise, the map in front of you will look like a random collection of foods, quirks, preferences, characteristics and conditions that are unique to you. Identifying these factors will enable you to create a more specific, personal weight-loss plan, one that you'll know you've put together by taking 'your style' into consideration.

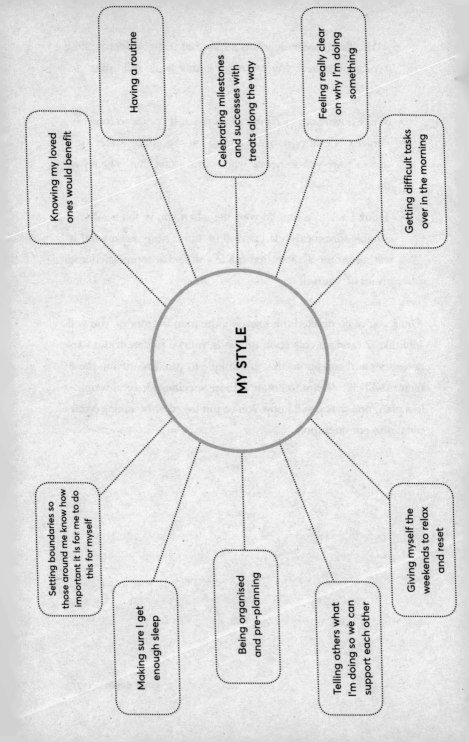

MY STYLE

- Having a routine
- Celebrating milestones and successes with treats along the way
- Feeling really clear on why I'm doing something
- Getting difficult tasks over in the morning
- Knowing my loved ones would benefit
- Setting boundaries so those around me know how important it is for me to do this for myself
- Making sure I get enough sleep
- Being organised and pre-planning
- Telling others what I'm doing so we can support each other
- Giving myself the weekends to relax and reset

what's good

Reframing problems as solutions

At the beginning of this process, I asked you to write a letter to yourself detailing all the things you don't like about not being where you want to be when it comes to your relationship with food and your body. I asked that you consider the negatives, which I imagine was relatively simple to do, since the thing people who come to me tend to have in common is that the negative impacts of their habits have, on balance, come to outweigh the positives. On many occasions, clients have come to me saying that they can't think of a single thing that could make them want to continue as they are, and that at this stage there are no positives.

Having delivered countless workshops during which I ask people to share the negatives associated with their habits, I can tell you that when it comes to weight loss, these tend to roll off the tongue and are pretty predictable. People explain that their inability to change makes them feel weak or out of control, that the foods they eat and the ways they eat them are causing their bodies to feel tired and unfit, that their self-esteem is suffering as a result of their body image. They express anxiety that their lifestyle choices will result in illness.

However, when I then ask people to share some possible *positives* of staying the way they are, responses take time and answers vary wildly. And often become personal, reflective, revealing and therefore very useful for the purpose of changing and replacing habits. That's because understanding what is keeping you as you are helps you to identify a need your current habit is fulfilling, or once fulfilled. What you see as a problem now was once – and may still be – a solution. If you take that solution away and the problem it was solving still exists, then you'll need to deal with the problem some other way. If you expect that to be the case, you can prepare for it, and put an alternative coping mechanism in place. In this chapter, you're going to uncover what's 'good' about your unwanted status quo, so that you can understand why you haven't been able to change already and put strategies in place for the needs that will crop up when you disrupt it.

I believe that any life change becomes easier to implement and sustain when we shift our focus from negative to positive in every possible way. We've already started to do this in previous chapters – for example, by shifting the focus from what your body can't do and hasn't done to what it can do and has done, you have been able to uncover useful motivational resources that you may have overlooked before. In this chapter, I will invite you to take this idea one step further. Following The Last Diet effectively involves treating yourself with forgiveness and getting to know yourself better. If you can understand why and how your unwanted patterns developed, you can take a more informed, understanding and compassionate approach to weight loss and address the very personal relationship you've developed with your body on your own terms, for the reasons that are most important to you personally.

Over the years when I was at my heaviest, a lot of people tried to remind me of the negative impacts of my eating behaviours, since bringing my attention to how 'bad' things had got was what they genuinely believed would spur me to change. Usually they would remind me about health risks, inform me of how many calories were in something I was about to eat, and remind me of how unhappy I'd told them I was with my size, as if these weren't things I already knew. I have no doubt that they were well intentioned, but the 'intervention' approach just never worked, because instead of motivating me to make positive changes, it made me:

- Self-conscious, because I felt exposed and observed

- Shameful and dishonest, because I felt judged

- Rebellious, because I'll change when I'm good and ready

- Defensive and patronised, because I'd been researching diets my whole life

- Disappointed in myself for still having this obvious issue that everyone could literally see, from my body size, was getting worse

- Hopeless, because even when I tried my hardest I couldn't imagine other people's suggestions actually working for me long term

- More convinced that people's main take-away about who I am was based on the size of my body

- Sad, and hungry for large quantities of foods that helped me escape that sadness as quickly as possible

As you can see, this combination of responses was not conducive to me getting motivated to like myself and find a viable long-term solution. I must admit that sometimes the odd scary lecture about my weight did cause me to lose some weight, but because it caused me to initially binge, then immediately starve myself for three days – losing maybe three pounds, nearly faint, and then binge again. As we discussed at the beginning of the book, I now know that things like spite, fear, revenge, anger and resentment towards ourselves or other people can get us going, but they don't keep us going. The same goes for changing for other people's reasons.

After years of listening to other people patronise me and tell me what's wrong with me, I now believe that even if it's someone's job to warn people about health risks, any advice should begin with things like, 'I imagine you already know this,' before saying things like 'you are dangerously overweight' or 'obesity is not healthy' or 'vegetables are good and biscuits are bad'. I just can't imagine anyone has ever gained the bespoke personal insight and motivation they needed to lose weight and finally keep it off after years of complex struggle by focusing on generic and obvious negatives.

Those who have spent years trying and failing to change their habits are more aware of the negatives than anyone else. They are living with those negatives twenty-four hours a day. They're constantly on high alert, listening out for possible options to get rid of those negatives. They've done the research, they have access to all the same information everyone else does.

Admittedly, there were some occasions when I was trying to lose weight or feeling particularly unhappy with my body, when I would go to people asking for practical weight-loss advice. Before I had the tools to gain proper insight into my own behaviours, I sometimes invited other people to tell me what they thought I should do. This was usually people I didn't know very well, probably because I hadn't had time to develop resentment around the content and delivery of their advice. I noticed that the people I struck off most quickly tended to do two things.

The first was to come straight in with patronising advice without asking for any backstory. They didn't ask what I'd already tried or wonder why I hadn't been able to maintain a weight I was happy with on my own.

It's a bit like spending four hours at home alone desperately trying to fix a laptop that's broken down. You've spent all afternoon frantically Googling every possible solution, called helplines, insurers and manufacturers, tried all the suggestions and nothing's worked. You've cried over lost work, been through a rollercoaster of hope and despair, and checked your bank balance to see if you've got enough to buy a new one. You've tried to see if you can borrow one from a friend in order to meet an important deadline and read all the forums and instruction manuals.

Just then, your partner casually arrives home, gathers there's a broken laptop situation and, without wanting more details, immediately assumes they can fix it. They sit down and smugly offer their miracle solution: pressing the reset button. While waiting for something to happen, they also take the opportunity to explain that you're in this position because you don't take care of things properly and remind you that you'll only damage it more if you don't change your ways.

They sit there, waiting for the laptop to come to life, genuinely expecting to have cracked it, and therefore completely believing that you've not yet considered this most basic of possible solutions. Because they never asked, they are oblivious to the fact that they walked in on you half an hour away from essentially graduating from laptop repair school. Does that sound like the kind of motivational support you needed, or the kind of support that makes you want to cry, eat a cake, and then cry again because the laptop's still not fixed?

The other kind of advice that eventually started making me switch off came from people who offered weight-loss plans that weren't sustainable long term because they didn't consider my mental health. They didn't care that I'd have to feel crap during and after the process in order to lose weight. The promise of feeling better as a result relied entirely on me being delighted about being slim. These plans were offered up by people who assumed that just losing weight would be enough to give me more self-esteem and sustain the resilience I needed to make considered choices with food for the rest of my life.

But I knew from experience that losing weight wasn't going to be enough to make me a happier person overall. It had never authentically increased my self-esteem in the past, so I had started to realise I needed something different. Experience had also shown me that unless I started feeling happier overall, I wouldn't be motivated to keep up any plan of change. Feeling miserable made me want to eat in ways that made me gain weight.

So, having established that we all know the negatives, I'm going to invite you to complete this next exercise either once or twice, depending on which approach makes sense for you. I needed to complete it twice – the first time to explore how it served me to eat the way I did, and again to explore how it served me to keep a layer of fat around me. It wasn't until relatively recently that I discovered there weren't only positives for me in how I was eating, but there were positives in staying overweight too!

This was a complete revelation to me. I discovered through the second optional exercise in this chapter that I had associated being overweight with getting attention from my parents from a very young age – even if it was attention because they thought something in me needed fixing. Staying overweight then became my excuse for delaying living life and avoiding taking risks and facing rejection; I'd decided that slimness was a prerequisite for these things, so that ruled me out. Before this realisation, if you had ever told me that staying overweight was serving me in any way, I wouldn't have believed you. That's the beauty of these exercises, they can help us to uncover the more subtle factors that drive our beliefs and actions when it comes to our bodies.

What's Good: Part 1

First, I'd like you to make a quick list of the main eating habits (or absence of eating habits) you believe are holding you back from losing and maintaining your weight. The general things you're doing or not doing with food that are making it difficult for you to achieve your goals:

1. _____

2. _____

3. _____

4. _____

5. _____

E.g. Snacking mindlessly in front of the TV, eating sugar when I'm stressed, prolonged bingeing after periods of restricting myself

Map: What's Good: Part 2

Now, in the centre of a blank page, write 'What's Good' and draw a circle around it. Then go to the first habit on the list you just wrote and ask yourself the following list of questions about it. On your map, write answers to any of the following questions that make sense for you, drawing a circle around each one as you go:

- What kind of comfort does it give you/did it once give you?

- What kinds of things does it allow you to do/has it allowed you to do in the past?

- What does it help you to avoid/has it helped you to avoid in the past?

- What does it make easier for you/has it made easier for you in the past?

- What does it protect you from/has it protected you from in the past?

- What parts of your life does it make easier to cope with/ has it made easier to cope with in the past?

- What does it help you feel more in control of/has it helped you feel more in control of in the past?

- What do you enjoy about it/have you enjoyed about it in the past?

- How does it connect you with others/has it connected you with others in the past?

- How does it benefit your relationships/has it benefited your relationships in the past?

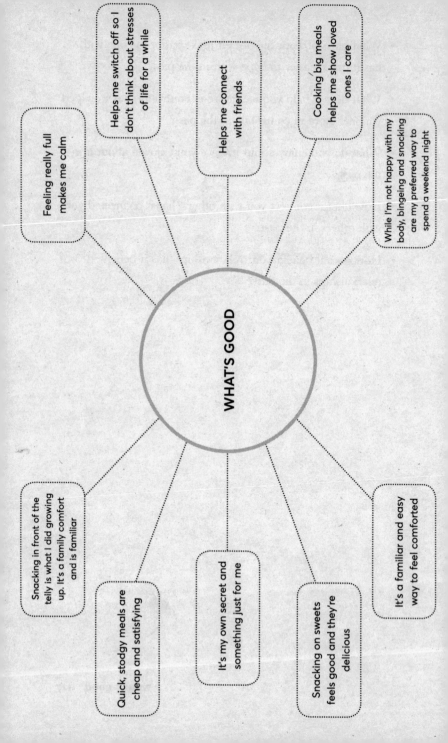

WHAT'S GOOD

- Feeling really full makes me calm
- Helps me switch off so I don't think about stresses of life for a while
- Helps me connect with friends
- Cooking big meals helps me show loved ones I care
- While I'm not happy with my body, bingeing and snacking are my preferred way to spend a weekend night
- It's a familiar and easy way to feel comforted
- Snacking on sweets feels good and they're delicious
- It's my own secret and something just for me
- Quick, stodgy meals are cheap and satisfying
- Snacking in front of the telly is what I did growing up. It's a family comfort and is familiar

What's Good: Optional Written Exercise: Part 3

If, like I did, you want to explore whether the forces pulling you to stay the same are multi-layered, then you can repeat this exercise with a different theme. In the centre of a black page, write 'What's good about staying this size?' and draw a circle around it. Then go to back to the first of the main habits you wrote down and ask yourself the following list of questions about it. On your map, write answers to the questions that make sense for you, drawing a circle around each one as you go.

Write down:

- The kinds of comfort it gives you to remain the size or weight you're currently at
- Difficult things that staying your current size helps you to avoid
- Things that staying overweight helps you to do
- Any comfort that being physically bigger gives you

When you've completed one or both of these maps, what you will have in front of you is a collection of the needs that you've identified are being (or have once been) fulfilled by the habits and circumstances you want to change. Now you have two questions to ask yourself:

1. Has staying the same way been solving a problem that doesn't need solving anymore?

2. Are your current habits solving a problem that still exists?

The people who will find this process the easiest are those who discover through the exercises in this chapter that they don't need their unwanted habits anymore. That they've outgrown their need for them as a coping mechanism; they simply hadn't stopped to acknowledge that before. A simple example is picking up the habit of eating a box of chocolates every night while getting over the sadness of a break-up. It's comforting and it serves a purpose in that moment. But then, over time, boxes of chocolate have found their way on to your grocery list, and you're still eating one an evening. It has subtly turned into a part of your routine, which brings with it associations and physical alerts and cravings. Then, before you know it, you're still eating break-up chocolate even though you're not heartbroken anymore.

If this sounds like you, then maintaining your weight loss will be much easier than it will be for many others. You can focus on simply repeating new habits as frequently as possible until they become your new norm, with minimal forces pulling you to maintain the status quo other than things like fear of change and short-term physical withdrawal.

If, however, you are in the category of people for whom their current eating habits are still serving a purpose, then there will be more commitment required to adopting new effective 'solution-habits'. The following exercise is designed to help you do that.

What's Good: Written Exercise: Part 4

In a notebook, copy out these sentences and complete them in as much detail as you can.

I see now that there are various understandable reasons I'm finding it difficult to change. These include . . .

_____

_____

_____

Staying as I am helps me fulfil some important needs, like . . .

_____

_____

_____

I'd prefer to be fulfilling these needs long term by doing things like . . .

_____

_____

_____

In the short term, I could distract myself from the discomfort of not having these needs met by . . .

_____

_____

_____

I hope that this chapter has given you any insight you may have needed to believe that you are not weak and there is nothing wrong with you. Your habits have developed for a reason, and whether you need them anymore or not, they're not 'bad' and neither are you.

testing times

Removing surprise where possible

It's time to start considering what, other than core beliefs from childhood, may contribute to the soundtrack of commands that tells you to go off track when trying to stick to a practical weight-loss plan. Forewarned is forearmed when it comes to triggers. So, we will now take time to reflect on the kinds of things that increase your desire to fulfil the needs you identified in the last chapter. If, for example, you identified that your current eating habits help you to deal with stress, then we need to assume going into a new plan that you will find it hardest not to eat in those ways in moments when you feel stressed.

Taking surprise out of the equation can help us to behave in a calm and considered manner when we're triggered. Later on in this chapter, you will complete a 'Testing Times' exercise which asks you to write down all the situations, states and conditions you suspect will make it difficult for you, specifically, to stick to a weight-loss plan.

We have explored some of the conversations we have with ourselves that can derail us. Many people, when they complete reflective exercises like those in this book, realise that it's quite a predictable set of conditions that trigger them to want to convince themselves to give up on their weight-loss plans. In the early stages of change, you will need to use past experience to pre-empt what might throw you off track and make you want to revert to the comfortable status quo.

Although I will encourage you to consider new reactions to challenging situations, you will no doubt be glad to hear that it will start happening naturally as soon as you begin to realise how predictable your patterns are. You don't need to have loads of tools at your disposal to be able to ride out short-term discomfort. The trick to responding in a way you're proud of is very often simply just expecting it. Expect the discomfort: expect physical cravings; expect to want to give up; expect to hear sabotaging self-talk and expect it to be difficult and scary sometimes – even if just for the simple reason that it's a change. If you can't avoid discomfort, then don't fight it. The important thing is to save your energy to withstand short-term discomfort, all the time reminding yourself why you're voluntarily choosing to withstand it. Ultimately, I want to show you how to welcome these feeling as an opportunity to practise getting through them without treating your body unkindly in response. Because once you have, you'll realise your own strength and find it much easier to stick to your plan.

Some of the feelings that will arise during this time you'll be able to predict, though some will seem to come out of nowhere. But the thing to bear in mind is that, inevitably, before your new habits have had the chance to become automatic, unavoidable and unforeseen circumstances will present themselves that make you feel like it's too difficult to stay on track. Although many of our triggers are out of our hands, how we react towards our bodies in response to them isn't.

When I am helping clients to stick to their weight-loss plans, I ask them to identify their high-risk scenarios, and I have noticed a few themes that keep coming up. Here's a list of day-to-day triggers that tend to directly or indirectly put people in high-risk scenarios where they feel more likely to lapse, especially during the early stages of change:

- Hunger

- Anxiety and stress

- Complacency

- Mountain-to-climb thinking

- Self-defeating, self-doubting thoughts

- Resentment – of others and the process

- Low mood

- Mindless use of smartphones

- Impatience and disappointment

Keep in mind, often we can overcome these in ways we're happy with when we're just dealing with one or two. However, when they pile up and present themselves all at once, we can find ourselves feeling very challenged indeed. That's why it's important to keep an eye on the levels of these things in general. To help us to feel like we still have resilience reserves in those moments when new things challenge us that we hadn't expected.

One of my clients described a situation recently where high-risk factors multiplied out of the blue, at an unprecedented rate, causing him to go from having no problem dealing with discomfort to going off track in a matter of minutes. He had gone to the supermarket after work to buy dinner and noticed that, having missed lunch, he was really tired and hungry. He recognised that the combination of how he was feeling and where he was meant he was in a high-risk situation. However, he told himself that he would use it as an opportunity to practise noticing the urge and pushing through it. So he focused on buying fresh ingredients as opposed to grabbing a family bag of crisps and eating them while he shopped. It had only been a couple of weeks since he started his weight-loss plan, but in that moment he felt in control and proud of himself in a way he hadn't experienced before. Almost smugly, he thought to himself 'I don't think shopping hungry is ever going to be a problem for me again.'

Just then, he got a call from his wife telling him that they'd be entertaining last-minute guests, who he happened not to be very fond of. This would mean he'd have to think of something else to cook because of their dietary requirements. He agreed and started thinking of options he could eat as well that would still keep him on track with his weight-loss plan. Before he had time to put his phone back in his pocket, he saw an email had popped up, informing him that he'd made a big error in a piece of work earlier that day, meaning he'd have to work into the night after the guests had left.

He put his phone in his pocket, looked up and saw someone who was slim happily working their way through a huge pack of crisps. He remembered that he hadn't lost any weight the previous week and started getting annoyed about the fact he had to have a plan at all; why wasn't he the kind of person who could just be naturally slim? Finally, he glanced at the lengthy queue at the tills and that was it. He called his wife and told her they'd be ordering take-out for everyone.

My client proceeded to spend the evening, following morning and week after that eating in ways that he'd identified as unkind and responsible for weight gain when he created his plan in the first place. His all-or-nothing thinking also meant that he neglected all the other habits he'd just started to get used to, having been on track for three weeks.

Now, I'm not saying he couldn't have still stuck to his plan. If he'd been further along in the change process, he may well have learned to say to himself, 'Yes, these things all make me feel like I want to go off-plan but they're not making me, so I'm choosing to disobey the commands they're giving me and hand myself over the version of myself that wants the best for me, the one who wrote the plan in the first place. Life will continue to look like this, it's up to me what I do to my body in response to it.'

But as it was so early in the process of becoming more self-aware about his patterns (plus he was in a supermarket), I'm not surprised the craving to relieve what began as just hunger went from manageable to unbearable in a matter of minutes.

Let's go back to our list of triggers and look at them more closely:

Hunger

This might seem obvious, but never underestimate the power of hunger. It can come on suddenly and lower resolve around food in a way you never imagined. It has a selective memory for how certain foods make your body feel. The commands it is able to create can be much louder than any of the helpful ones in your soundtrack. Hunger is highly skilled in convincing you that your plans are stupid. If you choose to create a plan that involves you being hungry at any point then, during the early stages of change, try to avoid taking that hunger to places that are filled with opportunities to go off-plan. Or at least take the edge off before. I've eaten many an apple en route to a dinner so that when it comes to giving the waiter my side order, I've lowered my chances of blurting out 'cheesy chips' when I genuinely intended to say 'salad'.

Another point on hunger is that it can cause us to forget how little it will take to make it go away and get us thinking rationally again. There were many occasions in the past when, shopping in the supermarket while hungry, I decided for one reason or another that I was going to lapse from a strict weight-loss plan, and because my commands were coming from hunger (and all-or-nothing thinking), I'd then purchase a buffet of foods to binge on. Enough to last me three days (thus creating an excuse to eat those foods for three more days so as to not waste them). It's wasn't until I'd take a couple of bites out of the first item in my bursting shopping bags that I'd realise how quickly my hunger was relieved, and that a healthier snack would have taken the edge off just as sufficiently – i.e. enough for me to start thinking rationally about what I was doing. At this stage I had the option of nipping my lapse in the bud after just a couple of bites and getting straight back on track. But a combination of never having seen myself be able to do that before and a passenger's seat full of all the foods I'd already bought meant that logic never stood a chance.

Anxiety and stress

Many of us experience stress and anxious thinking patterns to varying degrees at different times. Despite this, I have noticed that most of my clients come to me having never developed go-to coping strategies for them that can be used on the spot. Quite often, through exercises like the 'What's Good' map, clients discover that the habits that are holding them back from achieving their weight-loss goals are the ones that help them to deal most effectively with things like general anxiety and stress, so removing these presents them with some important needs that will still need fulfilling.

These days, I don't often tend to eat foods that are very high in sugar. That said, when I do eat them, I am immediately reminded how good they are at doing their job in that moment. If I'm feeling low, there is no denying that a delicious cupcake is going to give me a boost. That's fine. That's why, sometimes in response to feeling low, I choose to eat a cupcake.

But the cupcake isn't the only thing I can turn to. I can decide to listen to the ten-minute guided meditation app I have ready on my phone, or revisit a written exercise or run myself a bath. Now I know what you're thinking, none of these things are as effective as a cupcake. I agree, they're not as immediately effective, but they remain effective long term. They may not make you feel as good straight away, but they keep you feeling good for longer.

When an unwanted habit does a very important job for us, like relieve daily stress and worry, it's imperative that we respect that and acknowledge it for doing that, even if we want to change it. The kind way to create change for yourself is not to take away all the things that relieve you at once. Instead, start trying to reduce the number of times you go to those old habits for relief while increasing the number of times you turn to a new range of habits. Make sure your new habits are ones that you'd be proud to think of as your coping strategies for stress and anxiety in five years' time.

If you've identified daily stress and worry as resilience-lowering factors that have held you back from achieving your long-term weight-loss goals in the past, you may wish to complete the following exercise when met with them.

Optional Stress Exercise

Things that tend to cause me stress:

_____

How I tend to cope with this stress:

_____

How I'd like to be coping with stress in five years' time:

_____

Things I can start doing on a day-to-day basis that will help me get there:

_____

Things that tend to cause me to worry:

_____

How I tend to cope with worry:

_____

How I'd like to be coping with worry in five years' time:

_____

Things I can start doing on a day-to-day basis that will
help me get there:

_____

Like many of my clients, I have struggled a lot with anxiety in the
past, and the most effective coping mechanism I have found is
doing exercises, both physical and the written exercises in this
book. In fact, completing the written exercises often determines
whether I do the physical exercises.

After years of catastrophising and long periods of relieving
stress with food, I have learned to feel much more in control of
my actions when even the faintest signal of anxiety creeps in. A
large part of that is due to learning that when I take the worry out
of my head and take a second to write down the actual facts, I feel
immediately calmer. Don't get me wrong, as much as I wish it
could, I'm not suggesting that the following optional exercise I use
on myself will 'cure' feelings of general, day-to-day anxiety. What

it will do, however, is help you to collect factual data that you can't contest, which will show you how frequently you are spending energy worrying about things you can't change or don't need to.

Optional Anxiety Exercise

As soon as you feel anxious or notice that you've been in a cycle of worrying about the same thing for a period of time, stop, and make some quick observation notes, use your phone if that's easiest. The idea is that you quickly take a snapshot of what you think is going on in that moment and how you're feeling about it. Then, you put it away. It's effective for four reasons:

1. Having to stop for a moment and externalise can help you slow things down, focus your thoughts and give you a different perspective on the situation so you feel more in control of your response

2. The act of choosing to complete this exercise instead of responding as usual will remind you that you're investing in yourself and practising new ways of coping

3. Creating an ever-growing database of moments when you've felt overwhelmed allows you to revisit them – say a week later – to see how much needless, resilience-lowering worry you engage in

4. Over time, you will notice yourself making fewer entries because you've learned to 'cut to the end'. For example, when a familiar anxious thinking pattern crops up that

you've seen written down over and over again, you'll be more able to tell yourself things like 'I've worried about this a million times before and always landed on the realisation that worrying is not a useful way to spend my energy'

To try it out, simply commit to writing down your responses to these questions in the moments you feel anxious:

- What do I think is happening right now?

- What am I worried is going to happen?

Then, put your answers away and carry on as you were.

Over time, as your list gets longer and features some repeats, set a reminder in your calendar to check your worry exercise once a month for a couple of minutes, whenever you like. In that time, briefly reflect on your past entries. For each one, ask yourself with hindsight, 'Does my description of what was going on reflect the reality of what was really going on? And were my fears realised? If they were, was I better equipped to deal with them because I worried?'

Complacency

It might sound strange, but success can be a trigger for a lapse. I have seen people be caught out by it time and time again when it comes to sustaining new habits.

Often, I will spend a session with a new client discussing a particular event that they have coming up. One that is far enough away that they'd like to have started making changes by then, but not so far away that they will feel able to make instinctive food choices without going off track with their relatively new plan.

We will often play out high-risk scenarios and establish a plan of action. This in turn helps them to feel like they're going in prepared and that they've done the motivational groundwork to make decisions they will feel proud of after the event. I always warn my clients that creating a goal out of an event is only effective if you have considered how you will feel post-event. Sometimes after we achieve something difficult, we have a renewed motivation and resilience against the next challenge. Other times we feel we should be rewarded – often with the kinds of foods and behaviours that we were trying to change.

In other cases, clients fall into the trap of thinking that because they've found the first three weeks of their plan easier than they thought, when they have an event coming up, they don't need to give any prior thought to their food choices. That even if they eat something off-plan they've changed so much they'll be able to wake up the next day and be straight back on plan (even though that's never happened in the past). These clients tend to come back to me reporting that they had become complacent and completely underestimated the forces they were working against.

This process is designed to help you shift the way you think and behave in your everyday life in as many ways as possible, starting straight away. Plus, it's meant to make you feel better than before. But it's not a miracle cure, so however exciting and novel it is to be experiencing positive change across your life, don't forget that, when it comes to your body, you are trying to replace years and years of old habits. It's going to take a while for you to feel like you can do that without deliberately taking time to remember how important it is to stay on your own plan of change.

Mountain-to-climb thinking

This will be relevant to those who feel they want to lose large amounts of weight, or for whom it will take a longer period of time to reach their weight-loss goals, for whatever reasons.

I can't tell you the number of times I have thrown myself off track with otherwise successful weight-loss plans upon realising how far I still was from my ultimate goal. I've had people telling me I should do something about my weight seven months into very much doing something about my weight. Looking at a BMI chart and realising that despite weeks of hard work I was still months away from just about not being obese resulted in many a hopeless binge and quick return to old ways.

The most effective shift in thinking I have found to help with mountain-to-climb thinking is this: however many steps it takes to reach my goal, I'm going to have to take all of them at some point. So then it's up to me whether I want to take any of them more than once.

If it gets to week seven and you think, 'I've still got fifty weeks to go, what's the point?', then it can help to have the response ready: 'I want to lose weight eventually, and whether I get through week seven now or in three months, week seven is going to need to get done.'

Self-defeating, self-doubting internal dialogue and commands

We've covered this in previous chapters and we'll go on to look at all-or-nothing thinking patterns in the next chapter. If you feel that unhelpful inner dialogue plays a big part in you not achieving your weight-loss goals, then in addition to reflecting on and developing the 'My Soundtrack' and 'Cheerleading' maps, you may find it helpful to bring affirmations into your daily routine. A lot of people find the idea of this hard to get on board with, however, everyone I know of who's given it a proper chance for a few weeks has reported that it was genuinely helpful. For many who haven't done much personal development before, trying out this exercise will involve pushing past the cringe, going through the motions and seeing it as a harmless experiment. It still works even if you're sceptical while you do it.

First, choose a statement that directly challenges a common self-defeating thought you regularly have. One that you believe makes it harder for you to achieve your goals. You may want to refer to your 'My Body Can' and 'My Body Has' maps for inspiration here. Now, choose a short statement that firmly contradicts this self-defeating thought. To give you an example, if you're used to saying to yourself, 'I have no willpower and will probably end up failing at this plan as well,' then the statement you choose may be something as simple as 'I'm strong and committed.'

Then, you commit to saying this statement to yourself ten times every morning – privately, but out loud. (It can help when trying to make this practice a part of your routine to attach it to an existing daily habit. For example, you could do it in the bathroom right before you brush your teeth.)

'I'm strong and committed.'
'I'm strong and committed.'
'I'm strong and committed.'
'I'm strong and committed.'
'I'm strong and committed.'
'I'm strong and committed.'
'I'm strong and committed.'
'I'm strong and committed.'
'I'm strong and committed.'
'I'm strong and committed.'

While you do it, notice if any self-doubting thoughts or unhelpful dialogue creep in. You might start thinking 'this is silly' or be trying to think of all the times you've not demonstrated yourself to be strong or committed. That's OK, just notice what's happening and, if you feel you can, try to shift your focus to the times that have proven this statement to be true. The times on your 'My Body Can' map.

Different people experience different benefits from doing affirmations. The most effective role it has played for me is in helping to set something of a concrete intention for the day when it comes to how I speak to myself. So, if and when self-doubting thoughts come in, I'm reminded that I set time aside this morning as part of a mission to help me deal with this exact thing. It helps me remember that I can hand over to the version of me who wanted to try out the affirmation thing, the one who knows me the best today and wants the best for me tomorrow.

Resentment – of others and the process

For many years, when it came to eating, my mantra was 'I would rather be the kind of person who can eat whatever they like without gaining weight than win the lottery.' I spent my childhood wondering why other children my age stayed slim and I was getting bigger every day, when we were essentially doing and eating the same things. Like an angry stalker, I have observed the bellies of people who can consume huge amounts of food and continue to feel comfortable in their jeans. For various reasons, many of which I discuss in this book and many of which are out of my control, my body and mind did not develop in a way that resulted in me being able to naturally maintain a weight I was happy with. But some other people did. That would sometimes make me feel very resentful. And this in turn used to make me think, 'Why am I the only one having to worry about this? I should just face it: however hard I try this will never become easy for me. Maybe I'm just wired to be this way. This is pointless; I should just give up.'

Realising that, in the past, resentment had always moved me further away from achieving my goals helped me decide I would stop falling at this hurdle once and for all. Everyone has their challenges to deal with, this is just mine. And I'm lucky, because it's something I have the ability to change.

Gratitude can play a big role in helping with feelings of resentment too. Working in drug treatment, I've seen daily gratitude lists help people enormously with shifting the focus from what they wish they had to what they already do have across their entire lives on a daily basis. So I created my own version of a gratitude practice that many of my clients have turned into a very enjoyable annual ritual.

What I do is keep a jar next to my couch, filled with little strips of blank paper and a pen. When I think of something new I am grateful for – something that had happened that day, or as a result of something I'd seen in the news, for example – I grab a blank strip from my jar and note down it down. Then I just throw it back in the jar and forget about it. Provided I keep the jar in the right place, they collect without me thinking.

The positioning of the jar is very important. It needs to be somewhere visible and somewhere that you tend to be when you can spare (or be bothered to spare) thirty seconds to write something down. For me, this is next to the couch right alongside where I always place my mug of tea while I watch TV in the evenings. That way, when faced with the option of watching another advert or writing something nice on a strip of paper that's within reaching distance, I sometimes pick the paper.

Finally, on New Year's Eve, I tip out the jar and read through all the things I am thankful for that year. It's certainly a pleasant change from the many New Year's Eves spent focusing on what I don't have.

Low mood

Other than wanting you to feel as good as possible in every possible way because everyone deserves to, I want you to feel as good as possible, so that this process is as easy as possible for you. Creating your path of least resistance when it comes to achieving weight-loss goals involves considering everything you can independently be doing to feel more positive about yourself and your life.

When it comes to creating your practical plan of action, it is important that you factor in ways to take care of your mental wellbeing in general. It can be anything from including an action point to get more fresh air or connect with your friends more, to finally arranging a GP appointment for a counselling referral. Remember, change is difficult and it's a lot easier to do difficult things when you feel good.

Mindless use of smartphones

Many of us have got into the habit of looking at our phones to check emails, social media and the news before we've even got out of bed in the morning. This can leave us feeling overwhelmed and get our day started on an urgent, not very mindful note. Clients often tell me that viewing certain kinds of images on Instagram or being bombarded with WhatsApp notifications first thing in the morning can set them up to make less than kind decisions about how they speak to and treat themselves for the rest of the day. We are far better placed to behave in ways we're proud of towards ourselves and others when we feel we are on the best footing emotionally and physically. With this in mind, it can be helpful to try not to look at your phone until you've got out of bed, had a shower and eaten breakfast, for example.

Smartphone use is something that I discuss with a lot of clients when it comes to triggers. I have countless examples of clients tracing back steps to the beginning of a lapse and discovering it was triggered by something they saw on their phones.

I'm not saying that smartphones aren't incredibly useful. I suggest several times in this book that you can use your phone as a motivational aid. That said, many of us have developed a relationship with our phones that is not having a positive impact on how we speak to and treat our bodies throughout the day. It's often subtle and indirect, but it's real and I'm noticing it become more and more common.

Whether it's looking at unrealistic bodies and lifestyles on Instagram, reading harrowing news stories and angry threads on Twitter, getting absorbed in emails the second they've arrived in the inbox, feeling overwhelmed with bridesmaid group chat messages on WhatsApp, or developing an expensive online shopping habit, more and more clients come to see me intending to talk about food and leave realising they've spent most of the session talking about the things that happen on their phones.

If you feel that your relationship with your smartphone is distracting you from how you're really feeling, or that what you're looking at on it makes you feel less resilient or positive in any way, then it may be an idea to use your weight-loss action plan as an opportunity to introduce a new approach when it comes to your smartphone habits. The following exercise is one that my clients and I have found to be extremely effective. For those who have grown used to checking their phones last thing in the evening and first thing in the morning, this experiment may well provide a shocking surprise. The guidelines are simple: **Don't look at your phone for the first fifteen minutes of the day.**

By not looking at your phone for those first minutes of the day, you are deciding what you will expose yourself to. You're actively choosing not to start your day by exposing yourself to unhelpful content and messages that can get your day started on a negative foot. That first part of the day is your first opportunity to have a say in what kind of day you're going to have. Please don't voluntarily hand that power to literally everyone else in the entire world but yourself.

Some people will find this morning phone exercise much more difficult than others, not least because it involves keeping your phone completely silent and somewhere you can't see it overnight. Therefore, they can't fall asleep looking at it. Plus, the realisation that they're finding this exercise so difficult brings to people's attention how dependent they've become on their phones.

Persevering with this practice and collecting reliable data on how many times nothing bad happened as a result of you not looking at your phone is also useful in learning that many situations no longer need to be treated as an emergency. This shift in thinking of course becomes a transferrable skill when it comes to making challenging decisions around food.

Impatience and disappointment

We all want quick results when it comes achieving any goal that's important to us. When it comes to weight loss specifically, we are able to measure our progress in numbers and how we look. The problem comes when we measure our progress entirely on these things, because they are prone to fluctuate, and we don't want to base how motivated we feel on numbers. Plus, how proud of yourself you feel on a daily basis shouldn't depend on your body size or how much you weigh.

That's why, when you create a weight-loss plan, food and

exercise are just two elements of a much bigger objective: to treat your body with more kindness. That way, if you happen to weigh yourself one week and see that despite doing all the 'right' things you haven't lost any weight, you know that you're still making progress with your self-care and self-esteem routine and your personal development. All of your other habits are still moving you in the direction of weight loss, it's just a matter of continuing what you're doing until numbers on the scales catch up again.

I can think back to so many experiences when I've been totally on track until I made the mistake of weighing myself at the wrong time of the day (and month) and being left feeling disappointed and hopeless as a result. Feeling like this would often then lead to a binge (via a conversation with myself I didn't yet know I was having that went something like, 'My plan obviously isn't working, what's the point in going to all this effort, I'm basically in the same place I was a week ago, I may as well binge on everything I've managed not to eat, since evidently it makes no difference anyway.').

It can help to simply accept that your literal weight-loss process will, predictably, include boring periods of plateau during which it will be difficult to justify continuing to put yourself in challenging situations. At times your body will not do what you want it to as quickly as you want it to. Commit to remembering that so that when those moments do come around, you maintain an awareness that they were always going to, and that you've already decided you're going to push through them.

In my experience, it's soon after you push through the most stagnant sections of weight loss that you stumble upon the most rapid.

It's important to expect this process to be difficult. Exciting, positive, novel, but also difficult. Remember that you knew it would be hard and you've chosen to do it anyway. All the foods you may choose not to eat for a while are always there. Nothing is forbidden, you're just deciding to do this for yourself for a bit and see how it works out for you.

If, right at the beginning, I had asked you, 'How many points in the weight-loss process do you imagine are going be boring or difficult to push through?' I imagine you would have said quite a few. Remembering this can help you in those moments when it feels like you're not getting the results you wanted yet. If you'd have guessed that twenty out of sixty days would really challenge you, then when day five of challenge presents itself, you can think 'I expected this, and there's still more to come. I knew that it was going to be an inevitable part of achieving a truly meaningful goal.'

At the end of this chapter I will invite you to complete a map where you write down all of the situations, feelings, thoughts and circumstances that you feel directly or indirectly make it harder for you to stick to your weight-loss plan. First though, I'd like to introduce you to an exercise that you will be doing every morning. Stay with me, it's extremely effective and in total only requires five minutes of your time.

I started using this exercise to help me with weight loss, but I now use it every day to help me manage my behaviours in all areas of my life. It's become my version of a journal, and I spend just five minutes on it in the morning. I believe that this exercise was largely responsible for helping me push through in those weeks when I hadn't lost weight and wanted to throw in the towel, since it enabled me to realise that not losing weight was one of the predictable excuses I'd give myself to throw in the towel. It is based on the belief that simply expecting to be presented with a challenge is enough to stop you reacting to it in a way you later regret. It's also based on the assumption that you tend to fall at the same hurdles. Finally, it assumes that we all have moments when we look back on how we reacted to feeling internally or externally challenged and wish we'd handled it differently.

During the initial stages of implementing a plan of change, my clients often say that they wish we could start every day with a quick coaching session. Aside from this being unrealistic, it also goes against the spirit of handing over tools that people can use on themselves. But often it's not more tools that these clients want, it's a sense of accountability, a reminder that they've committed to something, and an opportunity to externalise their observations on how they're changing.

I believe that if you commit to completing the next exercise every day, and integrating it permanently into your routine, you will be able to provide this for yourself. When it comes to formulating your plan of change, you will be in charge of deciding what and how to eat and exercise. But I will insist that you include this daily exercise and treat it as seriously – if not more seriously – than the new food and exercise choices you make. It is designed to increase your moment-to-moment awareness of how you're feeling and become more aware of triggers, so that you can feel more in control of how you respond to them.

AM Check-in: Compulsory Daily Exercise

First, choose a time every morning (as soon as possible after you've woken up) when you know you can assign yourself five minutes to make some quick notes. Ideally, try to pick a time that you can add on to something you already know you do every single morning. That way you can create a new association. For example, the five-minute slot you may choose could be right after you get out of the shower, while you're drying off in a towel. I do my five minutes while I'm making and drinking my first coffee of the day. Make sure that you have some paper and a pen that works close to hand, so you don't waste any time or get deterred from completing it in the morning rush. If it's absolutely impossible for you to complete this on paper first thing in the morning, then it can be done on your phone during a commute, or even recorded out loud in the car as a voice note. The most important thing is that you repeat it every day and make it such a part of your routine that you notice when you haven't done it. At times when you want to skip it, instead get into the habit of saying to yourself, 'I deserve five minutes a day to check-in with myself.'

You are going to compile a list of the things that, if you had to put money on it, would directly or indirectly lead to you wanting to go off track with your weight-loss plan. All the circumstances and situations you're likely to face on that specific day that may test you. Anything from knowing there will be cake in the office for someone's birthday to expecting sugar cravings because you didn't get a decent night's sleep. That way, if and when those things present themselves, you've removed the element of surprise and feel more prepared to react in a way you're still of proud the next day. Sometimes, of course, this will involve not reacting at all. In these cases, the simple realisation of its predictability will help you to feel more in control.

So, from tomorrow, using the template below, start to spend that allocated five minutes thinking about as many possible triggers as you like, using whatever language is quickest and most comfortable for you. Once my list is complete, I take a quick photograph of it on my phone and then throw away the original – for added privacy and also so I have it to hand if I want to glance at it during the course of the day.

What might make it difficult to stay on track with my weight-loss plan today? e.g. Lunch with a colleague who always makes comments about my weight. Usually come away from those feeling crap and wanting to binge.

How I will respond: e.g. Remind myself that her comments aren't worth undoing all my plans for and make sure I look at the photo I took of my 'My Body Has' map for a boost on the way back from lunch. Remember that she doesn't mean badly and I'll regret it if I snap at her or get triggered.

What might make it difficult to stay on track with my weight-loss plan today? e.g. Leaving party at work, cake everywhere. Will be drinking so resolve around food likely to be low. Plus, I'll probably be hungry which never helps matters.

How I will respond: e.g. Eat a substantial lunch a little bit later so I'm not drinking on an empty stomach, stick to two glasses and remind myself that cake is available everywhere, I can have it whenever I want. I'm not forced to eat it because a colleague is leaving.

What might make it difficult to stay on track with my weight-loss plan today? e.g. I have to have a difficult conversation with someone and I feel really anxious about. Not sure breathing exercises and maps are going to take the edge off like a cheeseburger could.

How I will respond: e.g. Remind myself that this is an opportunity to practise my new skill of being able to watch the urge pass. I need examples of having dealt with this in new, kinder ways, and today can be one of them. I'll listen to myself want the cheeseburger and decide to let it just play in the background while I patiently wait for the dis-comfort to pass.

What might make it difficult to stay on track with my weight-loss plan today? e.g. When I have a slump as I always do at about 3.30pm and tell myself the only way to fix it is to eat chocolate at my desk.

How I will respond: e.g. Remind myself that it's never worked before and any boost that the chocolate gives me will be fleeting, leaving me feeling even more sluggish than I did before. If I do decide I really want some chocolate, reframe this trigger as a challenge to see if I can eat half the amount I usually would.

Once you feel more familiar with the check-in exercise, you'll find that you don't need such prescriptive questions. You may choose to extend the exercise to different areas of your life. So, in addition to pre-empting the things that make you want to eat in ways you're not happy with, you might also choose to pre-empt the things that tend to make you snap at a loved one or smoke cigarettes. Remember, pre-empting and externalising won't make the feeling of being triggered disappear, it will allow you to observe it as opposed to be driven by it. You will be able to collect examples of how discomfort also passes and evidence of how well you know your body and how predictable it is. Then, more and more often, for the rest of your life, when you feel discomfort, you begin to believe that it will pass and that you can endure it without adding to it by responding in ways you later regret.

My final word on the AM check-in exercise: I cannot stress enough how beneficial it is to commit to this practice every day. My clients who successfully incorporate it into their lives start seeing transformations in their behaviour more quickly than they could ever have expected. When it comes to keeping up weight-loss plans, they find themselves effortlessly jumping over hurdles that they fell at in the past. Trust me, if there's just one way you change your life as a result of reading this book, let it be that you make this check-in exercise a part of your daily routine.

Map: Testing Times

The time has come for you to create your own collection of internal and external high-risk scenarios, to enable you to become more aware of the warning signs and how they can pile on top of each other to create seemingly unmanageable situations.

First, write 'Testing Times' in the middle of a blank page with a circle drawn around it. Then write down the things that generally cause you have unhelpful, self-limiting and self-sabotaging conversations with yourself. Draw a circle around each one as you go. It may help to use some of these cues:

- Thinking . . .

- Doing . . .

- Seeing . . .

- Feeling . . .

- Discovering . . .

- Realising . . .

- Being exposed to . . .

- Smelling . . .

- Touching . . .

- Remembering . . .

- Convincing myself that...

- Saying . . .

- Hearing . . .

- Meeting . . .

A few final notes on triggers:

1. Everyone has their own triggers

2. New triggers will pop up throughout life, it's unavoidable

3. Triggers are important to be aware of when it comes to changing habits

4. Triggers can negatively impact how motivated you feel, physically and psychologically

5. Triggers do not control how you act towards your body – only you do

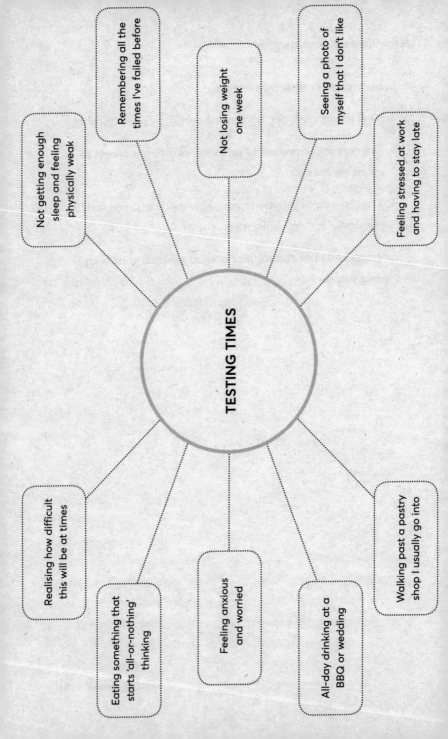

TESTING TIMES

- Not getting enough sleep and feeling physically weak
- Remembering all the times I've failed before
- Not losing weight one week
- Seeing a photo of myself that I don't like
- Feeling stressed at work and having to stay late
- Walking past a pastry shop I usually go into
- All-day drinking at a BBQ or wedding
- Feeling anxious and worried
- Eating something that starts 'all-or-nothing' thinking
- Realising how difficult this will be at times

gig's up

Don't insult your own intelligence

The excuses we make to delay starting something difficult and keeping it up can look irrational, illogical, even absurd when written down. Yet when they're just in our heads, they can compel and convince us.

We've discussed how we can throw ourselves off track with our plans by coming up with excuses that we use to sabotage ourselves. Self-sabotage happens for a number of reasons. These range from deeper things – like not feeling worthy of achieving success or subconsciously wanting to remain overweight for protection – to simply wanting to put off experiencing the initial period of physical withdrawal associated with changing your diet.

Regardless of why it's happening, sabotaging our own progress by allowing ourselves to be led by flawed internal logic has held back me and many of my clients from keeping up plans of change in the past. In this chapter, you will look at the common excuses that you make to justify going off track with your plans when things get difficult. We will build on the last chapter, where we looked at high-risk scenarios for going off track, but this time focus in on the stories we tell ourselves about the weight-loss process that don't help us and sometimes just don't make any sense. By starting to write them down, you will get into the habit of noticing – and challenging – their validity more frequently.

With hindsight, many of my clients identify that they fully relapsed with their weight-loss plans because two things happened to them in a moment when they felt challenged:

1. First, they believed illogical internal reasons and justification to go off-plan on one occasion

2. Then they threw the rest of the plan out of the window because of illogical, all-or-nothing thinking

All-or-nothing thinking is something I am very familiar with, but it wasn't until I started writing down examples of it in my own patterns that I realised how much I was letting it affect me. I've always liked to consider myself intelligent, yet when I saw the flawed logic behind the justifications I was allowing to guide my choices, I felt like a fool. When I did the exercise that you will complete in this chapter, I realised that six-day binges had begun with two thoughts that sounded something like: *It's raining so I deserve to 'cheat' tonight. That's ruined everything now, and the only day I can start again is Monday.*

I don't need to tell you that rain has nothing to do with what I eat; deviation from an eating plan does not 'ruin' the whole thing, and Monday is not the only day available for starting again. Yet I was guided by this kind of nonsense logic for years. If you feel that you too are readily suspending your disbelief for the self-limiting fictions you tell yourself, this exercise may help.

The next time you hear yourself making an excuse to neglect, change or ignore an element of your weight-loss plan, imagine the most intelligent person you know is standing in front of you. Choose someone whom you respect, someone whom nothing gets past, who is sharp and doesn't suffer fools gladly. Assume that they know how important it is for you to stick to your plan and they have your best interests at heart. Then, imagine justifying to them why you think you should go off-plan on this occasion, using your excuse as the 'pitch'. You will most likely conclude when you do this exercise that your excuse doesn't make as much sense as you once thought. Remember, you are also an intelligent person who is discerning and worthy of respect. You shouldn't suffer your own foolishness.

This exercise saved me in a moment when, despite being quite far into my weight-loss process, I was caught off guard by how suddenly tempted I was to follow a pretty ridiculous all-or-nothing internal command. I had ordered a take-out that I considered on-plan for me and my weight loss, which included a bottle of Diet Coke. They incorrectly gave me a bottle of Coke, in addition to a free starter and dessert that would have been off-plan. I put those foods to one side, but decided that since I was looking forward to a fizzy drink, it couldn't hurt to have one glass of full-fat Coke with my otherwise healthy meal. I had barely finished half my glass before I started telling myself that by drinking the full-fat Coke, I had ruined everything and that now I may as well eat the starter and dessert, which rather unhelpfully, had started to look more appetising than my meal.

However, having already done some self-awareness and mindfulness work, I caught my flawed logic in motion this time. I started thinking, 'Why does half a glass of Coke have to equal a binge? Do I really believe that is true?' If someone else came to me and said, 'I drank half a glass of Coke and someone told me it meant I had to sabotage myself with every choice I made after that for a while,' I would tell them not to listen to that person as they clearly don't understand even the basics of weight loss.

So, I decided to speak to myself out loud, and pretend I was talking to someone I know who has a very finely tuned bullshit detector, my old boss Ray Jenkins. I'd actually say things like, 'Hi Ray, so you know I'm trying to lose weight, well, I want to run something by you. I reckon I have no choice but to eat loads of fattening things tonight – and probably tomorrow, if I'm honest. The reason I have no choice is because I just drank half a glass of Coca-Cola. You'd agree that that's a good enough reason, right?'

Frankly, hearing myself made me laugh and feel a little bit embarrassed. Don't get me wrong, there are some foods that make you crave more of them physically, and that is a very real current to swim against sometimes. But in my experience, provided the all-or-nothing thinking is caught and curbed early, then any damage done in the process requires minimal effort to bounce back from.

In the past, I was most guilty of falling into the trap of believing my own excuses in the very first few days of starting a practical weight-loss plan. I've learned that this was also the case for many of my clients. What we shared was the habit of justifying going off track by telling ourselves it was still such early days that we may as well just start again tomorrow – i.e. nothing is squandered because we haven't lost any weight yet. Needless to say, this kind of thinking resulted in a succession of false starts that chipped away at our self-belief over time. All because we were so desperate to maintain the status quo and delay having to experience the discomforts of changing, we were prepared to believe stories that made no sense.

Committing to demystifying and myth-busting your all-or-nothing thinking can benefit you in many life areas, not least when it comes to maintaining your weight loss long term. That is because, treating your body well in every possible way will create conditions in which it simply doesn't feel right anymore to abuse it with unkind behaviour. That just doesn't fit in the new, kinder, day-to-day experience you've created for your body. This eventually makes it effortless to instinctively make better food decisions – i.e. the ones that help you maintain the weight that makes you feel most strong, attractive and healthy.

In order to create an environment in which unkind food and body choices simply don't have a place, you need to have lots of fingers in lots of self-care pies – just two of which are how you eat and how you move around. You can then challenge the kind of all-or-nothing thinking that reinforces an idea that your body isn't worthy of care, respect and enjoyment unless it is a certain weight or size.

If and when you fall off track with your eating or exercise plans, it will feel so much more natural to slip back into the new 'normal' you have created, not least because it's a nice place. It's a supportive place full of kindness, where you forgive yourself and continue to treat yourself nicely regardless of what you have or have not eaten. The bonus is that that this place of kindness just so happens to be one that gives you most resilience against all-or-nothing thinking and short-term physical cravings, which is of course what we need in order to limit any deviations from eating plans to harmless, enjoyable, intentional blips as opposed to catastrophes.

This myth-busting approach to the stories we tell ourselves can really help those who feel that they are living life 'on hold'. If you find yourself thinking things like, 'I'll pay attention to how I dress when I'm thinner' or 'I can't possibly start dating until I've lost weight' or 'I can't apply for that promotion until I'm a smaller size', then consider whether these things make any sense and whether debunking them is in fact a perfect opportunity to practise disassociating any of your value from your weight. Plus, doing things like taking pride in your appearance, placing importance on your social life and being ambitious in your professional life involves you doing the same kinds of things that create your kinder framework in which your kinder eating habits will comfortably sit.

Map: Gig's Up

We're now going to consider some of your own excuses and delay tactics. The ones that have, in the past, derailed your plans. Ones that make perfect sense at the time, but maybe not so much when you have to explain the thinking process behind them. First, write 'Gig's Up' in the centre of a blank page, with a circle around it. Then, write down:

- The excuses and delaying tactics you've allowed to work in the past to go off-plan with weight-loss diets when things got tough

- The excuses and delaying tactics you're already thinking of for this plan

- The excuses you're most likely to make to justify lapsing from your plan during the periods when you're not seeing fast results

- The excuses you're likely to make to justify neglecting the other self-care and self-development aspects of this process, like the written exercises and self-esteem building practices

You may find it helpful to finish some of the following sentences as a way to get the juices flowing. Although I still encourage you to think hard about your own collection of common excuses and stories, as they can be very creative and unique to you. (In the past, I used to justify a random binge when I was finding a weight-loss diet difficult because somewhere along the way I convinced myself this would actually speed up my metabolism by shocking my body out of a plateau and into weight loss.)

'Now isn't the right time to do this because . . .'

'It's not actually that important to do this because . . .'

'I should be able to make exceptions when it comes to things like . . . '

'_____ makes it impossible for me to change right now'

When you've finished, reflect on the collection of excuses that are currently clogging up your soundtrack when you try to make changes. Decide whether they look as convincing when they're written down. Even if some of them are reasonable, ask yourself whether it makes sense to let them impact your thought processes so much that you move further away from your weight-loss goals.

In the case of the excuses that make no sense, resolve not only to prevent them working specifically, but also not to let variations of them work either. I say this because when you start telling yourself that some excuses are no longer available to you, your mind may start to find loopholes, like, 'I lapsed because it was snowing, not raining. I never said anything about snow.' Commit to not insulting your own intelligence anymore.

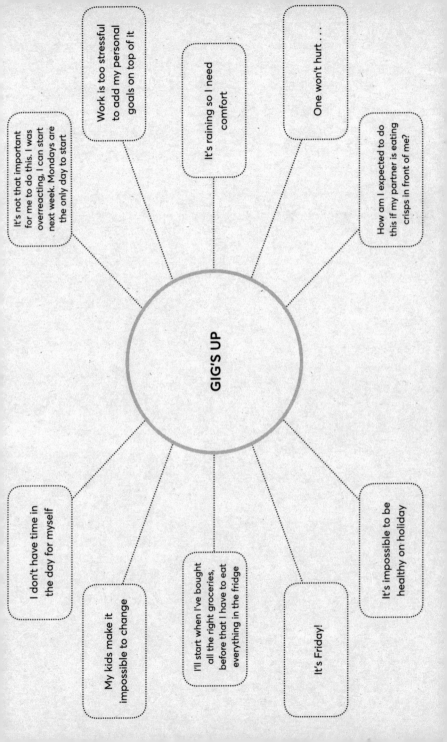

the plan

The time has come to plan what you'll
actually be doing to achieve your goals.

First, you will identify the 'off-track' behaviours and foods that you already know are currently contributing to weight gain or making it difficult to maintain a weight you're happy with.

Then you'll establish your 'gateway' foods, i.e. the foods that might even be undisputedly healthy but that you don't seem to be able to eat in moderation. You will decide whether you have faith in your ability to start behaving differently around these challenging foods or if – as part of this process – you will temporarily abstain from your 'gateway' foods as well as your 'off-track' foods. This can be revised and you may realise (as a result of your regular three-week check-ins) that you would like to cut these things out for a time, perhaps down the line, if not at first.

Later, you'll reintroduce all of the foods you want to eat in a planned, considered and mindful way, until you feel confident that you've developed new go-to habits. The idea is to make things as simple as possible in the short term and then create new habits to help you unlearn any core beliefs around some foods being 'bad' and others 'good.' Most importantly, you'll stop thinking you are being 'bad' or 'good' depending on what you choose to eat.

Once you've used the guidance in this chapter to create your first plan, you will get into the habit of reviewing it every three weeks until eventually you don't feel you need to tweak and reflect anymore.

The vast majority of clients I work with feel that they *do* need some eating guidelines in order to ultimately decide on a plan they can stick to without thinking about it too much anymore. They are tired of diets that are purely focused on losing weight as opposed to maintaining it, and want to create a bespoke, realistic 'way of eating', based on how their body specifically responds to tweaks in their diet over time. They are prepared to treat the process as an ongoing investigation until they've landed on something that works for them.

Temporary 'abstinence'

Perhaps you don't trust in your ability to eat smaller amounts of your off-track or gateway foods yet, because historically you haven't been able to. Or, the thought of not having to make any decisions about some foods at all for a while sounds freeing. Maybe you've been meaning to cut them out of your diet for good for a while. Perhaps, knowing yourself as you do, you'd prefer to avoid listening to the usual internal negotiations around certain foods for the time being and relearn how to eat them later down the line, once you have some practice under your belt, positive results and more self-belief.

Note: I know we've been told for years that it's not a good idea to cut anything out altogether, and I'm certainly not a nutritionist. I'm pretty sure though, that if someone decided they really wanted to stop consuming gummy bears or Coca-Cola for a couple of months – or indeed forever – they'd be fine.

Creating your plan

I believe that you already know what food choices are making your body gain or maintain unwanted weight, either because of what you're eating, how you're eating it or how frequently you're eating it. So first, I'm going to ask that you make a list of the foods you already know are making it difficult for you to lose weight. This can be for any reason, from the nutritional value they contain, what quantities of them you're used to eating, whether they're tied up in childhood associations or habitual patterns like snacking in front of the TV, how your body happens to respond to them, or any unkind, unhelpful internal dialogue they currently bring about.

I'm not simply asking you to make a list of objectively 'unhealthy' foods to cut out. It should also be a list of any foods that cause you to have illogical, self-limiting or unkind conversations with yourself. The foods that, for one reason or another, bring about guilt, all-or-nothing thinking and flawed reasoning which historically, goes on to dictate that your next food choice is an unwanted one. The foods that, when it comes to weight loss, for one reason or another, make you think 'I've blown it' when you eat them.

When it came to creating my own list of off-track foods to cut out in the short term, there were of course many obvious (and delicious) ones that I'd just never been able to eat in moderation or without feeling guilty and out of control. These were things like pizza, crisps, nuts, refined sugar and bagels. But there were also much less obvious foods that only applied to me, because of my unique relationship with them and therefore the specific unhelpful conversation they caused me to have with myself that threw me off track. For example, one of the foods I listed as off track in my first plan, without hesitation, was bananas. At some point during one of my many impractical dieting stints over the years, I apparently picked up the belief that bananas were a rebellious, 'bad' fruit that wasn't helpful for rapid weight-loss. I had only ever learned to associate them with eating five or six at a time, as they were often the food I'd initially lapse from a strict diet plan with in the past. So, when it came to creating an initial weight-loss plan for myself, I cut out bananas for a few months to keep it simple, and decided I'd reintroduce them when I felt ready to teach myself how to eat them using common sense.

Here's what the plan I'll be guiding you through will be comprised of. Once you've written it all out, you'll be ready to get going. You'll then keep reviewing this plan every three weeks and spending about ten minutes reflecting on how you got on with it. That's how you'll continually make sure it's moving you closer to your goals. If it's not, you'll work out why not and tweak and add to it until it is. Your plan table will be the basis of your three-week reviews and cover the following:

- Off-track foods and drinks

- Gateway foods and drinks

- On-track options (for breakfast, lunch, dinner, daytime and evening snacks, drinks - alcoholic or otherwise, take-out and restaurant choices)

- Quantity and frequency guidelines

- Feedback on internal shifts noticed, weight loss results, how you feel in your clothes, changes in internal conversations, general observations and any tweaks required to stay on track for the next three weeks

- Review date in three weeks' time (put it in your calendar)

After trialling various options with myself and my clients, I found three weeks to be the optimum time to review. It offers enough time to still see results (even if blips took place) plus it helps people avoid becoming obsessive with frequent weigh-ins. Ten minutes of feedback was enough time to notice weight-loss results, internal shifts, general observations about changes in the conversations happening internally and any tweaks required to stay on track for the next three weeks.

When I made my first plan, I made a really simple list in a table much like this one and eventually all the foods were in the right column.

OFF TRACK	GATEWAY	ON TRACK
Foods that I can't eat in moderation	Foods that make me tell myself I should eat the foods I can't eat in moderation	Foods that I can eat freely and feel I'm on track with weight loss

It took me eighteen months in total to lose eight stone. I spent the first four months losing weight quickly, mainly by staying away from off-track foods. I had fewer blips than I'd ever had before, and they were inconsequential thanks to my AM check-ins, excuse-busting motivational tools and, frankly, visible results. At around the five-month mark, I started noticing myself craving my gateway and off-track foods more frequently. Although I could manage the cravings, they were making me feel uneasy. After all, I'd never experienced losing weight while eating these foods. I worried that even tasting them again would derail me as it always had in the past.

So I decided to try reintroducing a couple of the foods that I was craving in a planned way. I chose the ones I felt had the least hold on me personally. I reframed the reintroduction of gateway foods as an exercise in busting myths about who I am and what I'm capable of. It became an exercise in creating a new relationship with an old friend. One in which I needed to establish – and adjust to – new boundaries and norms by being consistent in how I imposed them.

Admittedly, my first attempts at reintroducing gateway foods didn't go well. On a few occasions, I ended up eating a lot more than I'd intended and even *gaining* back a bit of lost weight due to gateway experiments gone wrong. But I quickly got back on track after each blip because I knew the experiments were responsible for the sudden weight gain – something that had never happened before.

Then something really amazing happened. When it came to reflecting on and reviewing the first plan that included the reintro-duction of gateway foods, I found myself feeling really positive about my progress overall! My main take-away was that I felt incredibly proud of myself and that I was noticing great shifts in my all-or-nothing thinking. Weight gain and experiment 'failure' or not, this was the first time I had ever demonstrated that I could get back on track after a blip. It was big for me! Over that three weeks of falling off track and getting back on without days, weeks or months of spiralling, I finally understood the power that my kinder internal dialogue had in helping me make decisions that move me back in the direction I wanted to be going. In the past, the combination of blips, lost momentum and weight gain after four months of steady results would have been more than enough to make me throw in the towel.

For the first time in my life, I cared more about how I felt about myself than how much I weighed. As a result, I felt worthy of giving myself the same advice I'd give a loved one: disregard the weight gain, tweak the plan so it's easier, refer to the 'My Body Can' map and stop weighing yourself so frequently. And that's what I did.

Logic and self-compassion had finally started to prevail. I couldn't believe that weight gain hadn't made me like myself less or beat myself up. I finally saw the process for what it was (a little food experiment that had caused a human body to gain a few pounds) instead of seeing it as evidence I was a weak person, failing and spiralling needlessly out of control. I genuinely didn't feel compelled to abandon all my other new acts of self-care because of numbers on scales. I realised that I knew too much about myself and about how motivating people works to go back. In the aftermath of each blip, I watched myself naturally want to do the opposite of what I would have done before. I actually *wanted* to practise forgiving myself quickly. I wanted to show myself that I could get back on track immediately. The work I'd done on developing my self-care, self-esteem and self-compassion in every area of my life had made it impossible to believe that I wasn't capable or worthy.

This realisation was enough to make the next few weeks far easier and the fact I didn't feel the need to eat away any feelings of shame or guilt around my weight gain certainly helped in a practical sense. I decided to keep the gateway foods in and try again. I kept trying and tweaking until eventually they didn't feel like gateway foods anymore. My usual patterns around them became predictable, manageable and eventually non-existent. I started transferring them to the category of 'on-track' foods. I simply learned, that if I did consume them, I should expect to want to eat more even past feeling full. I could expect to tell myself I could ride out unhelpful urges and become more and more conscious of how much I was eating of them – and how frequently I could eat them – in order to maintain a weight I'm happy with.

After some time experimenting with myself this way it was very smooth sailing to lose the rest of my unwanted weight. I'd started mastering the art of seeing a challenging situation around food as an opportunity for personal development. As I became more confident in my ability to choose how I speak to and behave towards myself, I was able to overcome bigger and bigger challenges with ease. By month eleven, when it came to creating a new three-week plan, I was in the habit of moving four or five off-track foods into my on-track plan each time. Usually I wouldn't even choose to eat them despite 'allowing' myself to, as I now had so many new options that I enjoyed more and made my body feel better. When

I did choose to eat previously off-track foods, whatever they were, I stuck to each new set of guidelines without trying too hard. That's because all the kinder, bullshit-detecting, impulse control skills I'd been practising throughout this process were transferrable to every food and every circumstance. I was now convinced of my own abilities and there was no turning back.

By around month fourteen, I stopped needing to do check-ins or weigh-ins as frequently. I noticed that I seemed to be able to effortlessly, consistently and spontaneously make decisions that ultimately aligned with my long-term goals. I just made sure I kept doing my daily AM check-ins and applying my self-kindness tools at every opportunity. As I started approaching the end of my weight loss, I had developed a habit of treating lapses or blips as enjoyable experiences. I'd stopped regretting them, even if they were unplanned. All the three-week plans I reviewed and created had eventually come together to create my 'way of eating', my Last Diet. Thanks to my experiences with gateway and off-track food experiments as well as the new curious, respectful and compassionate approach I'd adapted to my body's needs, I found myself instinctively knowing how much of certain foods I could generally 'afford' to eat and how frequently I could afford to eat them.

Table: Populating Your Plan

Choosing your off-track foods

First you'll establish what you won't be eating at all, at least for the first three weeks of your weight-loss plan. Think about the foods you've never been able to eat in moderate quantities. Next, think of the foods you currently eat that you know for sure are contributing to weight gain, because of how frequently you eat them and how your body responds to them. There might only be a few foods and drinks that you choose to list, or you might start with more and review them as you go along.

In a notebook, write the heading 'OFF TRACK', and under it, make a list of the foods that, for whatever reason, you don't currently think you're able to enjoy while being able to lose weight.

Choosing your gateway foods and drinks

When we're used to all-or-nothing thinking and believing our own internal negotiations, it's not uncommon to go off-plan as a result of a technically harmless decision that eventually turns into a lapse onto the foods we're trying to avoid all together. For example, as I mentioned earlier when I was populating the gateway foods section of my plan, that you are about to fill out, too, it included bananas. Not because I thought they were contributing to my weight gain as obviously as things like pastries and pasta binges, but because I still considered them 'bad'. My ingrained crash diet, all-or-nothing thinking associated them with being off track. They'd never been allowed on my usual extreme diets, so I knew that if I consumed them, I'd start thinking 'I've blown it' and convince myself that I should eat the off-plan foods while I'm there.

With the exception of foods that specifically make us crave others, gateway foods are very personal because they're often based in our associations rather than with common sense principles of nutrition and weight loss.

By choosing to adopt The Last Diet, you're acknowledging that you're choosing to start losing weight but you haven't yet truly addressed the issue of not being able to make common sense decisions around some foods.

Now, write the heading 'GATEWAY FOODS AND DRINKS' and under it, list the foods you think cause you to have self-sabotaging conversations or crave off-track foods.

Choosing your on-track foods, meals and drinks

To do this, first consider your realistic needs. Perhaps refer to previous maps you've completed that remind you of what sort of plan works for you.

If you're a person who likes to snack throughout the day, and don't want to change this habit now – or ever – then cool. Just reflect on what points in the day you usually snack and list possible alternatives that you believe are more helpful in helping you lose weight. If you can't think of any, put aside twenty minutes and do some online research.

About 90 per cent of my clients and workshop attendees don't find they need to do any initial research to get going on their first few three-week plans. Seasoned dieters have a lot of knowledge, both about their bodies and the healthier alternatives that they don't mind substituting their unhelpful snacks with, provided they just give it a bit of thought. If you don't trust that you'll eat them in reasonable amounts, then set yourself a simple quantity guideline.

Even if you have a lot of experience and knowledge, I strongly encourage you to make an ongoing habit of looking out for new foods and recipes that you consider on track. Ones you can imagine wanting to eat when your task is to maintain your lost weight. The ultimate 'way of eating' you eventually create will need to be realistic, enjoyable and varied. So, even if you can manage to lose weight for six weeks with only two snack options on your eating plan, it's worth anticipating boredom. Commit to keeping your plan interesting, not least as it's an investment in establishing how you want to be typically eating in the future. When it comes to reviewing your plan every three weeks, consider whether all the food options you gave yourself were appealing enough and whether you're growing bored of them yet. If you are, commit to some research and consider yourself on a mission to create the most varied list of options you can.

Apply exactly the same thinking to breakfast, lunch, dinner, take-out and restaurant options. Take some time to list all the options you have available to you as on-track foods and meals. Ones you know you can enjoy and still feel like you're moving towards weight loss. Think back to any previous weight-loss attempts that worked, at least for a while, and write down any of the meals you enjoyed cooking and eating as part of them. Write down all the possible options you can think of. Again, if experience of dieting and your body's usual responses to foods isn't enough, then absolutely do some research for undisputedly healthy recipe options. If experience has taught you that low-carb diets tend to make you feel good, then research which one of those seems most sensible and look at the food options there. If the basic formula of calories in and out has served you in the past, then research what low-calorie recipes seem appealing. If you know you don't want – or don't have time in the morning to eat a substantial breakfast – then look online to see if there's a healthy smoothie you can make.

Ultimately, I can give you all the guidance and templates in the world. But in order to make realistic changes to your current 'way of eating' that you can sustain, you'll need to view this process as an experiment for a while. Practically speaking, the thing that makes this your Last Diet is that you're conducting an ongoing and comprehensive enquiry into what choices make your body specifically gain and lose weight. I believe that the vast majority of people reading and relating to this book already know what general type of diet tends to suit their bodies, and what they'd need to Google for recipe options that enable them to lose weight.

Setting quantity and frequency guidelines

If you think that things like portion size or the frequency with which you tend to eat on-track foods could still contribute to you gaining weight, you can create some additional guidelines. You might find it helpful to create your own rules, like 'only on weekends' or 'half the amount I usually eat' or 'not if I've had pasta for lunch'. If you think this would be helpful for you then either add your 'rules' after each on-track option, or in a new column of your table.

Note: although we want to keep internal negotiation at bay with a few clear rules on how much you intend to eat, being able to follow general, default eating guidelines spontaneously is the ultimate goal. You may feel that you initially need more specific non-negotiable rules around what quantities of certain foods you're allowed to eat. That's fine.

Three-week reviews

Every three weeks, spend ten minutes feeding back on your plan. Reflect on how things have gone and record your progress so you know what updates you might need to consider. If you haven't achieved the results you expected, use this time to write down why you think that may have been the case. Identify the choices you made over the last three weeks that you suspect are responsible for this, and decide what tweaks to make. Perhaps you could look at adjusting the portion sizes of some foods you know are technically healthy, but that you suspect aren't helping you with weight loss goals. You may change the frequency with which you're allowing yourself snacks, and consider researching more weight-loss friendly alternatives.

If you realise your first plan was too difficult, just tweak it! Compassionately and curiously observe why the plan didn't work for you and go again, this time creating more manageable guidelines to start with. You should feel that every three weeks, no matter what you weigh, you're embarking on new experiments with enthusiasm. That's because you know that this time, instead of investing in a quick fix, you're completing a total mind and body audit. You're investing in understanding your specific needs and what choices are best for your body at this stage in your life.

When you're finished recording your progress, add the date of your next three-week review to your calendar.

From abstinence to moderation and mindfulness

There may be some foods you've cut out that you don't want to eat again. That's your call. Most of the people I've seen lose weight successfully don't like the thought of never eating their off-track foods again. That said, after weeks, months or even years of not consuming those foods at all, they're very apprehensive about trying to eat them again, for fear it will slow down their weight loss or cause them to gain unwanted weight. This is very rarely due to the calories, fat or carbs they fear these foods contain. It's almost always because they still don't have specific evidence of having eaten these foods in ways that still enable them to lose or maintain weight. Even if they've seen great shifts in their mindset and ability to choose common sense principles in challenging moments, they've not practically seen themselves undo their all-or-nothing ways when it comes to certain foods. Abstinence has taught them how to not do something. It hasn't taught them how to do it differently.

For that, you need to see evidence of having done it the new way over and over again consecutively, until it gradually gets easier and eventually becomes your default way. How long this takes to happen will vary enormously from person to person, depending on anything from how things look for them when they start this process to how many opportunities they have to practise undoing old habits.

My clients tend to want to reintroduce off-track foods when one or all of these things happen:

1. They've achieved their weight-loss goals and feel ready to maintain their weight

2. They miss their off-track foods and want to reintroduce them in a controlled way

3. Regardless of where they are in the process, due to a boost in their self-belief and the priority of finding a long-term 'way of eating', they feel ready to start practising new ways, even if it means they risk slowing down their progress in the short term.

Creating your reintroduction plan

The next time you're due a three-week review, simply choose a couple of your gateway foods, and add them to your list of 'on-track' foods. When it comes to deciding what quantity of them you'll be attempting to eat and how frequently, create guidelines that you imagine you'll have to follow in order to maintain your weight once you've lost it.

This approach works even if you're reintroducing gateway and off-track foods before you've lost all the weight you intend to lose. That's because, as your three-week reviews will have shown you, as you lose weight, your body will require tweaks to your plan in order to keep losing it. In this way, one of the simplest ways to define your ideal quantity and frequency guidelines when it comes to reintroducing gateway and off-track foods is to start making the decisions of someone who is tasked with maintaining a lower weight. Essentially, when you set guidelines for what new habits you want to create around challenging foods, you'll be taking a guess. You'll base this guess on how you suspect this food will need to need to feature in your life if it's to stay around in some capacity, but not cause you to gain unwanted weight.

When it comes to your AM check-ins, make sure that you focus your contingency plans around attempts to reintroduce these new foods. However motivated you may feel, remind yourself that now more than ever, it's important to commit to expecting things to get difficult and reminding yourself that you're capable of doing difficult things.

When you get to the next three-week review, reflect on how things went, just as you've done before. Make notes on your progress in your ten-minute feedback exercise.

If you managed to stick to your new habits around previous gateway foods, but still gained weight or didn't continue to lose weight as you'd hoped, ask yourself why you think it was. Do you suspect the guidelines around them need to be tweaked so that you're consuming less of them or eating them less frequently? If you're keen to keep enjoying and practising on these foods in particular, would it make sense to tweak the guidelines on some of your other on-track foods? If you've reintroduced chocolate twice a week, it may be an idea to take the take-aways down from twice to once a week. Again, it's all a process of experimenting with your choices and capabilities and observing how your body and mind respond with compassion and curiosity.

If you didn't manage to stick to your new guidelines around gateway foods, or you found it more challenging than you feel ready for, then either simply try again or move them back into the off-track category again for now. I suggest you base the decision of whether to move a gateway food back into the off-track category on how many consecutive times you managed to behave differently around it. You're the only one who can really judge when you're ready to test yourself, so if you feel like you're getting closer to being able to keep up the new guidelines consecutively for three weeks, then go again! Carry them over. I know this may feel like a risk, but, the way I see it, if you adopt the principles of The Last Diet and believe in your ability to get back on track however the experiment goes, you can afford to take risks. You can willingly put yourself in front of consecutive challenges in a conscious effort to make them less challenging.

The idea is that you continue reviewing this same template every three weeks until you've found your new 'way of eating'. How long that takes will depend on how much weight you want to lose, how much of this process you embrace and a range of other factors. The most important part in making sure this is a long-term sustainable new 'way of being' is that you notice shifts in your self-belief and self-esteem.

You continue to gradually introduce gateway foods at three-week reviews, until your list is more varied and you've grown skilled at adjusting quantities and frequencies so that your overall food intake balances out to help you achieve your goal of losing or maintaining weight. When you feel more comfortable around all your gateway foods, you will start introducing your off-track foods and keep applying the same tweaking review process. So you include them as on-track foods and set yourself guidelines based on how you logically guess you're going to need to be eating them in the future if you're to maintain a lower weight.

Committing to AM check-ins

When you know what your off-track foods and food-specific new challenges are going to be, you can make your five-minute AM check-ins more specific. You can spend that five minutes guessing what kinds of things will make you want to eat off-track foods that day and deciding how you'll respond if and when you're met with that challenge.

I strongly believe that when it comes to building the self-awareness, self-belief and internal bullshit-filter you'll need to make changes that last, the daily AM check-in is the most effective and useful habit you can adopt.

Physical exercise

I don't profess to know much about fitness, but when it comes to acknowledging the benefits of moving my body around, not only to manage my weight but also to feel good in every way, we're in no-brainer territory.

That said, I think it's important to make an admission in the spirit of complete honesty – though I hope you will not let it influence your decision if you are in a different position to the one I was in when I lost weight. The thing is, I really hated exercise. I hated being out of breath, every minute feeling like it was lasting a lifetime – and actually every single thing about it from the mirrors to the running shoes to the Lycra to the yoga mats to the 'burn' and the elusive 'zone' everyone kept going on about. I was not an active child, or teen, or young adult, or adult-adult, and I had never found a way of moving my body on purpose that I enjoyed. The fact that it was usually either in a state of extremely full or extremely starving certainly didn't help matters.

I discovered in hindsight, having completed exercises like the ones in this book, that I could trace the source of many of my unsuccessful false starts in part to starting to exercise as soon as I started changing what I was eating. It appealed to my all-or-nothing, dramatic-transformation-wanting thinking style at the time. Plus, it made sense, since exercise aids weight loss both in a literal sense and through things like effectively relieving the stress and anxiety that can lead to unkind food choices.

The problem was that, for me, in the initial stages, exercise was a trigger to want to behave in ways that threw me off track with my eating choices, and therefore actually delayed me from achieving my weight-loss goals overall. To make matters worse, since I only associated exercise with feeling uncomfortable, embarrassed and disappointed, not to mention physically exhausted, I used to use exercise as an excuse to go off track with my eating plan for weight loss. I often fell into one of two thinking patterns:

1. I've done exercise, that means I've been good and so I deserve to 'cheat'

2. Exercise has left me feeling crap and wanting to change that feeling by binge eating

The only point I ever saw in moving around on purpose was to aid weight loss. I had no experience of it being useful for much else. And certainly no experience of it ever being enjoyable in itself. The closest I'd ever got was on the rare occasions when I'd enjoy that euphoric (and smug) feeling afterwards.

Now, I know that I could have been easing myself in from day one by doing things like getting off the Tube one stop early on the way to work and walking the rest of the way, or trying out a gentle exercise class that wasn't created with weight loss in mind. I could have downloaded free five-minute guided workouts on my iPad and, just once a week, done a little routine.

But no. The way I thought before, if I was going to exercise, I needed to be training for a marathon or already slim and just trying to keep it up. The old 'just take the stairs instead of the escalator now and then' stuff didn't fit into my extreme, quick-fix, boredom-fearing kind of thinking. As far as I was concerned, taking the stairs twice in a week wasn't going to make me lose weight and so there was no point feeling out of breath. It didn't occur to me that the more frequently I did it, the less out of breath it would make me, and that the reverse was also true. It didn't occur to me either that every day doesn't exist in isolation when it comes to my choices. That they all add up, regardless.

I realised that I was in fact getting more unfit every year, despite increasing the number of fitness programmes I'd signed up to every year. Looking back now, I always knew deep down that my all-or-nothing logic when it came to being more active was flawed. I know that because if someone I loved had come to me fifteen years ago and asked whether small changes adding up is a better long-term strategy for their body than a series of extreme false starts, I would have given them the kind advice. I just wasn't applying the same wisdom and consideration when it came to how I thought about and treated my own body.

I am delighted to report that I eventually started becoming more active. I'd like to say that's because I wanted to be, but it's not. In fact, it was because my body just felt stronger, more capable and easier to move around. I naturally felt more connected with it and its needs because I was finally paying attention to what those needs actually were. For the first time it felt like we were a team and I started wanting to see what my body could do. Surprising myself with the new eating habits I was managing to keep up made me want to start surprising myself in every other way, not least in ways that might speed up my weight loss.

Perhaps it was because my body was unfamiliar with exercise, but it responded quite dramatically to making my day even just a little more active. The things I decided to do had to be really easy, so that I would want to keep them up and repeat them enough times for them to become habits. When I finally gave the 'quantity not quality' approach a go, the results were amazing. By choosing tiny little missions throughout the day, I was able to measure how quickly I could see progress. This progress in both my fitness levels and the amount of weight I was losing convinced me I needed to give more organised exercise a chance again.

Now, I can tell you, hand on heart, I truly love the feeling of being generally active in everyday life, as well the process of organised exercise and of course the feeling I get afterwards. I have found ways of exercising that suit me, and ruled out ones that don't. I would even say I look forward to exercise these days. I now know what people mean when they say they are going to 'blow off some steam' with exercise. In fact, I have pretty much disassociated exercise from being something I do to help me remain slim. First and foremost, it's become one of the most effective methods I've found to improve my mental health.

I'm telling you this because it's an example of how quickly you can undo years of presumptions about yourself and exercise. If, five years ago, you had asked anyone who had known me for any amount of time whether they considered me physically active in any way, other than when I was answering the door to the pizza delivery man, they'd have said, without any hesitation or doubt, 'No'. Now, if you ask those same people and the ones who've met me in the last couple of years whether they consider me to be a fit, active and, dare I say, sporty kind of person, they'd say, without any hesitation or doubt, 'Yes'.

You too can change any self-limiting beliefs and decide on purpose 'what kind of person' you want to be when it comes to your physical fitness. There are a few pieces of advice relating to exercise that I wish I had known or believed sooner. I have recorded them below in case they are useful for anyone else who wants exercise to be part of their lives but has no experience of sustaining that in the past:

- All physical discomfort isn't bad. Trust that your body will tell you if you're about to have a heart attack

- Feeling out of breath is normal and gets better much more quickly than you expect

- Doing exercise you don't like is a false economy

- How great you feel after exercise is often related to how much you invest during exercise

- When it comes to choosing an exercise you want to take up, make it something you like the idea of getting better at

- Don't feel guilty about caring how you look when you exercise. If fancy gyms and buying new gym gear help you exercise more, then do it. You're investing in your body

- Other people aren't judging you. And even if they are, you have a much more important thing to be focusing on – yourself

- Don't make presumptions about what benefits you should be gaining from exercise. Just go through the motions as best you can for as long as you can. Your body will start showing you benefits you never expected

- Exercise can be a form of meditation, and not just in the obvious way, as with practices such as yoga. If you happen to feel most present, connected with your body and free of thought when you're in a dark spin studio with disco lights, doing highly choreographed, high-intensity exercise with dance music and motivational speeches blaring, then do that

- This 'zone' people brag about getting into is real. And trust me, you want some of it. It's so effective at helping you stop thinking that you don't even realise you were in it until you've left it. Don't go looking for it though, it'll find you as soon as you've gone through the physical motions enough times

- You don't have to exercise early in the morning for it to be useful. If you don't want to have to blow dry your hair before work or miss out on sleep to be fit, you don't have to

- Don't overload yourself with other people's opinions about what exercise you should be doing. Stick to the basics at first and learn to be guided by what your body is telling you makes it feel good overall

- Don't pre-pay for unappealing exercise plans offering miracle results assuming you'll learn to love them. You won't want to go back enough times to learn anything, and you'll be out of pocket

- Allow yourself to keep trying out new things and expect to keep changing your mind about what you want to be a fixture in your routine. Explore and experiment with every new type of exercise you can, in as many different settings as you can, before signing up to anything long term

- If for some reason you do choose to wake up early to exercise in the early days when you're still finding it difficult, try going to bed in your gym gear the night before

- Don't use progress with exercise as a measure of how well your weight loss is going. Make weight loss and maintenance a bonus. Remember that if you focus on exercising to improve your mental fitness, your body will naturally start taking care of your physical fitness

I will now invite you to consider what physical activity you might like to include in your plan of change. If, like me, you would prefer to address food first and bring in 'organised' exercise later on in the process, that's fine. But please learn from my mistake of associating all physical activity with pre-planned exercise by identifying how you can be more active in even the smallest of ways throughout your day.

Adding exercise to your three-week plans

Feel free to simply include a commitment to exercise in each of your plans. Review how you found each experiment as you do with food, and, if you find it useful, give yourself some more prescriptive guidelines to stick to.

You can use these enquiry questions for some inspiration.

- In what simple ways could I be slightly more active in the mornings?

- In what simple ways could I be slightly more active during my working day?

- In what simple ways I could be slightly more active during the evenings?

- What types of exercise would I like to start doing right away?

- What type of exercise that I already do would I like to continue doing?

- What types of exercise would I like to take up at some point?

- What types of exercise could I be excited to get better at?

- What types of exercises could I do that are designed to target the body areas I most want to work on?

- What types of exercise do I think would leave me feeling most invigorated?

- What types of exercise do I think could benefit my mental health?

- What types of exercise could enable me to enjoy active time with my loved ones?

- What types of enjoyable exercise could I plan to do during the weekends?

- What kind of physical activity can I do regardless of weather conditions?

- What kind of physical activity can I do to increase how much fresh air I get?

- What types of organised exercise would realistically fit into my routine?

- What time of the day does it most suit my body to exercise?

- If I try to imagine the type of exercise routine that I could maybe be convinced I'd keep up long term, what habits would it need to include?

Note that, in keeping with the spirit of The Last Diet, creating actions to improve your physical wellbeing extends to all aspects of your body. As such, if completing exercises like these makes you realise, for example, that in order to take up tennis again you'll finally need to make that appointment to get your back pain sorted, then be sure to make that an action too.

When the three-week reviews end

Eventually, a shift will take place that enables you to avoid the chore of planning. Naturally, when this is will differ from person to person.

Even though it took me eighteen months to lose all the weight I wanted to, at around month fourteen I noticed that I could gradually do my check-ins less and less frequently. I had got the hang of balancing out my choices and the habits that caused me to lose the last couple of stone are pretty much the same habits that helped me maintain the weight I was ultimately happy with. Many people reading this book will feel they can reduce the frequency of their check-ins long before I could. Either because they have much less to lose, or because they don't have as much investigation and unlearning to do. I grew to love my check-ins, as they punctuated my progress and reminded me that I'm investing time in diversifying my list of enjoyable food options. Ten minutes every three weeks was totally doable and fun.

If you commit to your AM check-in exercise and focus on your overall personal development, you'll naturally find yourself needing to be far less prescriptive when it comes to ensuring you make sensible decisions about food quantities that work for you. Things will get easier – and stay easier – when you start realising that your goals are being achieved with the help of an eating plan, not because of one. You will start respecting your own intelligence when it comes to excuses you'll accept for going off track. You'll be able to acknowledge that you're having to make difficult decisions and already be in the habit of reminding yourself, first by glancing at a map and eventually by just knowing, that you're capable of overcoming much more difficult challenges. You'll be in the habit of catching any unkind, unhelpful messages you're giving yourself. You'll be practising your new impulse-control skills daily and collecting examples of moments when you've been able to treat an urge as an alert, instead of a command. You'll be in the habit of reminding yourself that you always have a choice of what action to take when you're triggered in any area of your life. You will have gathered evidence of being able to stop a lapse in its tracks and challenge flawed thinking patterns once and for all.

If you commit to backing yourself long term by developing these habits, and simply seeing food plans as an aid for moments when common sense and trusting yourself aren't enough, the results can be transformative. The Last Diet process believes that it doesn't matter how many delicious on-plan meal options you assign yourself, there will be moments when you'll want to go off track, and that ultimately, no book is going to stop you from doing whatever you want. There will be moments you hadn't planned for, when you have to make a call. In order to feel empowered in the actions you take in those moments (and the ones you take straight after them), you ultimately need to trust and believe in yourself more than you trust and believe in any plan.

This process is not about controlling what you eat. It's about believing in your ability to apply common sense principles and not treat urges as commands. It's about exploring what foods stop you losing weight and teaching you to think differently about them until you can meet them head on and still trust that you'll make the best decision for you. And more importantly perhaps, trust that when you don't make the ideal choice, you have the ability to immediately make the next choice the best, most kind, most logical one, however difficult it may be. Once you've mastered this, a shift will take place that can benefit you in every area of your life. You'll then feel less need to keep planning.

Again, it will happen at different times for different people, depending on how things looked for them when they started this process. But when it happens, when you truly start believing in your ability to treat an urge as an alert instead of a command and become prepared to call yourself out on the spot, you won't need a plan to write down how many cashew nuts you're allowed to eat in order to still feel you're on track with weight loss or management.

Plan and review guidance

Now it's time for you to start working through your own plan using the guidance throughout this chapter and the maps you've created along the way. To recap, first you'll recreate a table like this one for yourself, either in a notebook or on a computer.

OFF TRACK	GATEWAY	ON TRACK	[OPTIONAL] FREQUENCY/ QUANTITY GUIDELINES

Then, when it comes to your first check-in, you'll simply sit down for ten minutes (or more if you like) and reflect on this table as well as your AM check-in exercises and decide what the next three weeks of your plan are going to look like.

It might be helpful to consider incorporating the below prompts if you find that you need a little more structure in your observations. Again, these are just suggestions. Feel free to word this however suits you best and add anything you feel would be helpful to each plan.

- I will complete my check-in at __ AM everyday

- I will put aside thirty minutes, every three months to reflect on my check-in exercises and update my 'My Body Can' and 'My Body Has' maps

- What elements of my plan aren't helpful/sustainable?

- What tweaks will help make my eating plan feel sustainable long term?

- What is the combination of food, exercise and check-in habit actions that make up my new and improved plan?

- What habit actions make up my new 'normal' way of eating?

- What habit actions make up my new 'normal' way of being physically active?

And there you have it. For now, it might be an idea to do something nice for yourself, however small. Whether this chapter took you two hours or two weeks to complete, you deserve serious acknowledgment for the time and energy that you've put into creating a plan that affects what you do all day every day.

bring it on

If life is going to be filled with challenges
that make us stronger, why not choose
what some of them are going to be?

Through my work in addiction, I have discovered that when it comes to the question of how best to manage high-risk situations when we're in the process of changing habits, there are two main schools of thought:

1. Focus your planning on avoiding triggers, as decreasing the frequency of exposure to risk will logically decrease the likelihood of unwanted lapse

Or,

2. Assume you will be around triggers all the time, so be aware of them, but focus more of your energy on building your self-belief to deal with unexpected ones

The Last Diet approach very much supports accepting, expecting and preparing for triggers. It's not that I don't think we should always be on the lookout for ways to minimise our experiences of stress or upset. But the way I see it, learning to better manage our overall wellbeing should be a lifelong, ongoing process. So, if you've identified that the eating habits you want to change are currently helping you manage stress, and you want to start to lose weight before you've developed effective long-term coping strategies for stress, then you should accept that you will probably feel more stress during the first stages of changing what you eat. And you're going to need both short- and long-term strategies for dealing with it.

That's why I think that when you feel strong enough – and only then – you should start to reintroduce some situations and circumstances that you enjoy but find it difficult to keep up your weight-loss plans in. Later in this chapter, you will complete an exercise to help you identify and prepare for these situations.

We can decide to accept that our plan of change will initially involve unpleasant things like annoyance and hunger. We can choose to not only prepare for these things if and when they crop up, but also use them to our advantage. We can reframe them as opportunities to fast-track the resilience-building process.

When I took time to reflect on which weight-loss plans I'd tried weren't right for me, I noticed many shared the characteristic of requiring me to feel in control of both my internal and external environments at all times in order to see results. These plans helped me lose weight, but in order to keep it up and keep seeing results, I had to create a protective bubble around myself since I always felt so deprived and ready to pounce at the first sign of a trigger. In my case, this meant isolating myself and staying indoors with only my (often tasteless) designated 'meal' to entertain me.

It just goes to show how much less I liked myself back then, because it's difficult to even imagine putting myself through that now.

While I know that some people strongly believe in avoiding facing high-risk situations in habit-change at every cost, it personally doesn't work for me because:

- It makes me feel like I'm just holding old habits at bay, as opposed to shedding them entirely

- It makes me feel like I can't trust myself to make the right choices in challenging and unforeseen circumstances

- It stops me having fun that I'd rather have with a bit of compromise as opposed to not have at all

In this chapter, you're going to draw from your 'Testing Times' exercise to create a collection of high-risk situations you will not only overcome, but you will attempt to welcome when they inevitably arise as an opportunity to practise your new skills and strengthen your resilience and self-belief. Overcoming the high-risk situations you do have some control over helps you to believe in your ability to overcome the ones that pop up out of nowhere.

I've often noticed those who are in long-term abstinent recovery from alcohol addiction to have notably high levels of resilience against temptation to relapse. It appears, though, that it's not in spite of alcohol being everywhere, it's *because* alcohol is everywhere. When it comes to sustaining motivation, repeatedly exposing themselves to the substance they are desperately trying not to consume can actually make it easier. I've gathered through conversations with those in long-term abstinent recovery from alcohol addiction that it's because they grew so aware of why they shouldn't drink, and had to remind themselves of the preferred life they're moving towards so often, that they just cut to the end and stopped even seeing having a drink as an option, let alone a temptation. Because alcohol is everywhere and associated with so many occasions, they had plenty of opportunities to practise showing themselves that they could be around it without consuming it. By committing to building their resilience, connection with their bodies, self-belief and self-awareness, over time they have desensitised themselves to it and made their peace with their default, automatic choices, safe in the knowledge that when they decided not to drink again, they had their own best interests at heart. This also meant that they felt they could still feel strong in situations where alcohol was around – or even appeared unexpectedly.

When I recently asked a client in long-term abstinent recovery from alcohol addiction how she managed to resist all the shelves of booze every single time she went grocery shopping, she told me:

> After hundreds of successful trips now I just instinctively know that some sections of the supermarket have things I don't need and that I know full well I will never need again. I was already used to thinking like this, not just because I've never needed nappies before, but because I'm lactose intolerant. I just told myself that another allergy I've discovered is the one I have to alcohol. It has side effects that are dangerous for my body and mind. So, the alcohol section is not for me and never will be.

No point debating about it, negotiating with myself is a
waste of time. I just get on with the rest of my shopping
and walk straight past it now.

This is how I'd like you to feel when it comes to how you approach
weight management and unwanted food choices. Like you can cut
to the end with your internal dialogue about why it's important for
you to stay on track, and not feel like anywhere is out of bounds
for you just because you could be exposed to triggers. I want you
to feel like you're in control of how you behave regardless of
where you are and what challenge you're faced with because you
know yourself and you've laid strong internal foundations. Again,
planning is of course important, and as I've mentioned before, just
pre-empting triggers can be enough to make us change our
response to them. But we can't always anticipate them and we will
never be prepared for every possible risky scenario. We're better
off doing what we can to make them less risky scenarios and eventually not risky at all scenarios. Plus, we don't want to spend our
energy constantly trying not to ever become stressed or hungry or
tired or in the company of someone irritating, or in the company
of onion rings. This only reinforces the idea that our actions are
at the mercy of these things, which they absolutely are not.

Coming back to alcohol, the focus of my work has more recently
shifted to helping those who don't want to stop drinking, but who
do feel they have a drinking problem and that they need a general
plan to stick to. A 'way of drinking' that they'd never taken time
to create on purpose. Those who succeed in doing this are
extremely inspiring to me. That's because they're the ones I can
relate to most when it comes to learning how to eat a human-sized

portion of something I've only ever been able to eat a bear-sized portion of. I had to create my first 'way of eating' thirty-odd years after I began eating. I understand what it feels like to be around my substance of joy, comfort, protection, relief, distraction and despair all day, and constantly need to make new decisions about how you're going to behave around it. Abstinence from food is not an option (although at some points I've wished it was), so I have to see, smell and handle my substance all day every day for the rest of my life.

The clients who are successful in implementing alcohol-management plans long term seem to share something with those who are successful in implementing weight-loss plans long term: they frequently have to be in high-risk situations they can't avoid.

A common example of this is a parent whose weight-loss plan involves not eating the much more enticing food they have to prepare for their children. This gives them a number of opportunities to strengthen their resilience every day. Eventually when they push through it enough consecutive times, they stop associating the children's food preparation with their own and realise they've stopped feeling so powerless at these times.

During a period when I was receiving weekly counselling, I noticed that I came away feeling prouder of myself when I'd reported to the therapist that something negative had happened – and I had responded to it positively – than when I reported than nothing negative had happened at all. This happened enough times until the things I initially defined as negative events stopped coming up at all, because I hadn't even had to think about how I responded to them anymore. My new habits had become automatic ones, and so my triggers had become less triggering. That's what the exercise in this chapter will begin to help you to do for yourself.

It may sound silly, but these days when I'm met with internal or external challenge, I try to feel grateful for it. More and more every day, across every possible life area, I have committed to reframing challenge as an opportunity to practise my new strategies and have more say in what my soundtrack sounds like. I know that if I want to be 'the kind of person who can easily eat half a portion of popcorn and leave the rest', then I need to have shown myself that I can do that as many times as possible. If I want to be the kind of person who, when anxious, exercises instead of reaching for chocolate, then I need examples of having done that over and over again. Of course, I am presuming common sense tells you here that I don't recommend you intentionally making yourself feel anxious to practise easing it with exercise – you can wait for that trigger to find you. But becoming a slightly more frequent cinema-goer in order to collect more examples of when you managed to eat half of the popcorn isn't such a bad idea.

Written Exercise: Bring It On: Part 1

When it comes to keeping up your new eating plan for weight loss, what current high-risk situations for lapse would you like to eventually become low-risk situations?

1. _____

2. _____

3. _____

4. _____

5. _____

6. _____

E.g. When I'm hungover, when I'm stressed at work, on Friday night, in a restaurant, after a row with my partner, when celebrating my success, when I've got my period

Map: Bring It On: Part 2

Now let's use this information to create a map. First write 'Bring it on' in the centre of a blank page, with a circle drawn around it. Then, use each item in your list above as further headings and circle those too, being sure to leave space under them for more notes.

Now, for each scenario, try to guess how many times you'd need to have responded to this situation in the way you want to in order to truly believe it's not a high-risk situation for going off track with a weight-loss plan anymore. Essentially, to genuinely believe you've changed. Then draw empty tick boxes under each heading, one for each occurrence. (Though if it's something like 100 times then you may want to just write 100 and commit to drawing yourself seven new empty tick boxes a week until you hit 100.)

The idea is not only that you boost your self-belief by recording your progress and achievement, but also that you start to get excited about practising your new responses – whether that's responses to challenges you put yourself in front of on purpose or those that present themselves out of nowhere.

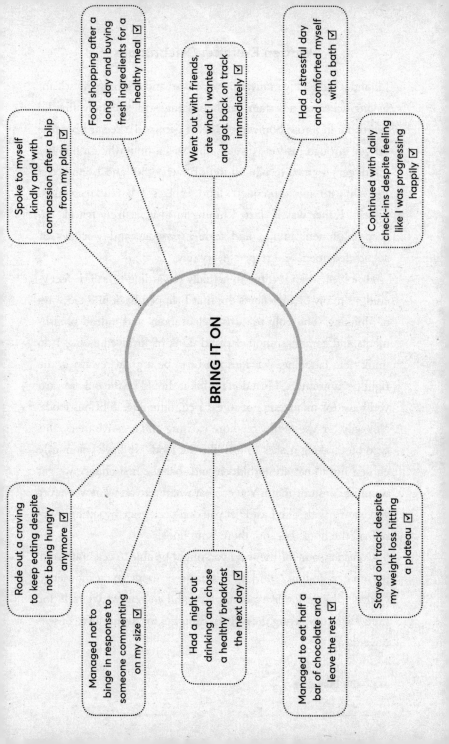

BRING IT ON

- Spoke to myself kindly and with compassion after a blip from my plan ☑
- Food shopping after a long day and buying fresh ingredients for a healthy meal ☑
- Went out with friends, ate what I wanted and got back on track immediately ☑
- Had a stressful day and comforted myself with a bath
- Continued with daily check-ins despite feeling like I was progressing happily ☑
- Rode out a craving to keep eating despite not being hungry anymore ☑
- Managed not to binge in response to someone commenting on my size ☑
- Had a night out drinking and chose a healthy breakfast the next day ☑
- Managed to eat half a bar of chocolate and leave the rest ☑
- Stayed on track despite my weight loss hitting a plateau ☑

Written Exercise: Celebrations

I found it incredibly motivating to reward and celebrate myself for having ticked off a certain number of high-risk situations that I'd overcome in a row. Sometimes I felt I deserved a reward because I'd got through just one (usually this was a time when a number of triggers seemed to pile on top of each other and I handled it so well with my subsequent food choices I barely recognised myself). Either way, I started tuning in to what truly felt like an accomplishment to me and feeling prouder and worthier of acknowledgment and respect every day.

However, when it came to actually rewarding myself, I discovered, as many of my clients do, that I slipped back into old ways of thinking. The only rewards, celebrations and indeed punishments and commiserations I could think of involved eating. I do think rich, fattening, delicious food can be a great reward in the right circumstances, I just don't think it should be the only reward you have for managing not to eat rich, fattening, delicious foods. Not only are we worthy of more exciting and creative treats, this type of thinking makes us feel like the foods we have voluntarily chosen not to eat are forbidden and that the first chance we get we must consume them. You can eat whatever you want whenever you want – with The Last Diet you don't celebrate by letting yourself off the hook, because there is no hook.

Consider some of the ways you might be able to celebrate your personal milestones during this process (both to acknowledge yourself things for like pounds lost and to reward yourself for things like completing the written exercises for twenty-five consecutive days).

Write some suggestions of rewards and celebrations here:

1. _____

2. _____

3. _____

4. _____

5. _____

6. _____

E.g. Take a long candle lit bath, take myself to the theatre, treat myself to a massage, spend a Sunday in bed reading magazines, invite a friend out to raise a glass with me, buy myself some flowers

A final note on this chapter: even if you are quite far into your change process, if you don't feel comfortable with the 'putting yourself in front of stuff on purpose' idea, then just don't do it. Focus on building your resilience in preparation for the high-risk situations that come out of the blue. Then after you've dealt with them, log them on your 'Bring It On' map and/or your 'My Body Can' map.

damage control

It's not damage when you know
how to get back on track

This chapter will help you feel more equipped to get back on track from any blips as soon as possible. It builds on previous chapters which explain that there is a step we often overlook when it comes to how we behave towards ourselves when met with challenge.

To recap, in short, a 'lapse' is a planned or unplanned deviation from your 'on-track' general 'way of eating' that you can bounce back from quickly.

I would argue that if you adopt The Last Diet completely in the spirit it's intended, you will never consider anything a 'relapse' again, long term. That's because you won't see starting again practically as a false start anymore, rather as a signal that you need to review your plan more before it's perfect for you in the long term.

You know by now that eating and exercise make up just two of the many elements of The Last Diet. By the time you've attained your default way of eating, 'lapses' will just be the moments you choose to enjoy foods or ways of eating that you know aren't helpful for weight management before immediately going back to the ones that are. Provided you keep demonstrating to yourself that you can immediately bounce back to your default 'way of eating' without letting these lapses drag on, they will stop being lapses and start being your version of 'eating everything in moderation'.

Perhaps in the future, you'll realise that, for whatever reason, you've neglected your practical weight-management habits for a few weeks, perhaps because of a holiday. Maybe that's caused you to gain some weight. That's fine! If you still complete your AM check-ins, go back to your self-defined best 'way of eating' to manage your weight and how you're generally treating your body and mind with more kindness than you did before, then you're still on track with many of the important parts of The Last Diet.

One of the main challenges when changing habits around food is that we are exposed to food and food decisions all day every day in a range of different contexts which may well keep changing for the rest of our lives. Those of us who are highly skilled at negotiating with ourselves internally and finding reasons to go off track are simply given too many opportunities to make unkind decisions, full of technicalities and get-out clauses. That's why, when it comes to weight loss, we're better off trying to challenge flawed logic across all areas of our lives than focusing on food specifically. Even if you get a huge tattoo across your hand that says 'YOU KNOW THOUGHTS AND FEELINGS CAN'T FORCE ACTIONS', there will still be moments in the future when you choose to keep that hand in your pocket.

That's because before the bounce-back tools can work, you have to want to use them. You have to want to remind yourself that all-or-nothing thinking doesn't make sense, and that your plan is really important to you. You have to *want* to put steps between feeling an urge to do something you'll later regret and actually doing it. Sure, sometimes it feels as simple as:

High-risk situation = relapse

But in reality, it's:

High-risk situation + internal conversation = lapse
then
Lapse + internal conversation = relapse

There have been many occasions when my clients have pushed against The Last Diet's requirement to shine light on their excuses and question the validity of their internal justifications. As I often say, this is because they don't want to give up their 'fuck it'. They know deep down that their excuses and delay tactics make no logical sense. They know hunger pangs don't take the wheel and drive their body to KFC. But they don't want to give up that mindless but comforting option to escape from discomfort by allowing themselves to believe their own excuses. So they choose to keep their 'fuck it' as a security blanket.

Think back to one of those moments in the past when you've impulsively gone off track with a challenging diet plan. A time when you felt so desperate to give up that you threw in the towel and quickly binged on a vast buffet of foods you'd felt deprived of. You'd white-knuckled it through the tasteless meal choices but a bad day at work meant you finally just said, 'Fuck it'. Now you're slumped on the sofa post-major binge, feeling that horrible kind of full you'd forgotten about. The one that makes you feel physically sick and somehow still hungry at the same time. Would that moment have been the kind of time when you'd have wanted to go find a relapse management map to complete? Would it be a period of time when you'd be feeling really resilient against self-sabotaging thoughts?

Say you have plans to eat at a restaurant, and when you arrive you're starving and very angry at someone close to you. You already looked up the menu online beforehand and decided on what you'll order. It's a meal you're really looking forward to, as it's delicious but also keeps you on track and doesn't make you feel deprived or restricted. However, when you arrive at the restaurant, you're informed that the menu has changed. So much so in fact that now there isn't a single thing on the menu you can eat to keep you on-plan completely. Now you have to choose whether to remind yourself of what you know you should do, or simply revert easily into your old habit of using 'being caught out' as an opportunity to order yourself enough food for three people.

When thinking about what you'll do when faced with these sorts of dilemmas, even if 99 per cent of the time you made the kinder decision, the other 1 per cent can throw you off track. If that's combined with all-or-nothing thinking styles, then the 1 per cent can throw you off track for a while. You won't always *want* to tune in with your thoughts and bodily sensations enough for your excuses to become undeniably unconvincing.

So, what can we do to make it difficult for even that (very ambitious) 1 per cent of times to throw us off track for long? We can commit to designing the best possible environment in which mindful acts just make sense and mindless, unkind ones just don't. It's more obvious how to start creating these conditions externally.

Say, for example, you're months into your plan and you've developed a repertoire of recipes you're happy with and that align with your chosen 'way of eating' long term. You're weeks into an exercise routine and have friends who turn up every week to do that with you. Your check-ins have become part of your day-to-day routine. You've introduced kindness into your morning and your fridge is packed with healthy breakfast options. Everyone around you has grown used to seeing you take more pride in your appearance and care more about yourself in general. You're absolutely convinced now that self-sabotage only delays things and that you're in control of your actions.

But one evening, for a variety of different reasons, you decide to flick the 'fuck it' switch with your eating. However, you wake up in the morning and, whether or not you have the energy in that moment to challenge unhelpful thoughts, your entire life is already challenging unhelpful actions. You already have plans to meet your friends and exercise. You already have a new outfit you're looking forward to wearing. From the moment you get out of bed, you're performing kind actions for yourself. You have actually made it easier to carry out your plan than try to revert to old ways. In fact, going back to old ways requires much more effort on your part than getting back on track. There would be too much arduous and unwelcome undoing to be done.

As well as setting a more fitting scene in which to live, all those kinder habits dotted throughout your day are playing an important role in keeping planned and unplanned lapses from becoming relapses ever again: they are imposing friction. In that, they are creating as many speed bumps as possible between thinking about throwing in the towel and actually managing to do it.

Some speed bumps are of course choosing referring to your maps for the support and reassurance you need, or just opting for a short-term delaying tactic. But the real strength ultimately is in our default routine, which provides the infrastructure to get us back on track in those inevitable moments when we simply don't want to care, while our thoughts catch up.

We can use this 'speed bump' thinking in a range of ways when it comes to riding our short-term physical cravings during the initial stages of change. For example, if your plan includes not ordering take-aways from your phone anymore, don't just delete the app. Sign out of the app, after deleting your pre-filled payment and delivery details. Create more and more speed bumps; more effort required to follow through on your impulse to act; more steps to take between an idea and its execution. Even if you've logged back in and decided what to order, perhaps while you're looking for your credit card you'll catch sight of what you're doing and decide to stop that unwanted lapse in its tracks.

One great way of imposing a speed bump that requires no administration is simple delay tactics. Tell yourself that you have every intention on acting on whatever impulse that you want, but that you'll try to wait for thirty minutes before you do. When it comes to impulses to eat urgently in ways we quickly regret, imposing a delay can make all the difference. That's because very often when we've reassured ourselves that our guaranteed fix is available as if we need it, we feel more able to calm down, slow down and to try a new, healthier approach before we resort to it. Because of both the changing and usually fleeting nature of physical cravings, by the time it comes to allowing ourselves the fix we wanted, more often than not the urge has passed.

Removing speed bumps can then help us when trying to create new habits, especially in the early days of change. As soon as you think of a new kinder habit you'd like to make part of your routine, do everything you can to remove barriers between wanting to and doing it. I do this all the time and find every day that just a tiny bit of speed bump-flattening in advance can go a very long way.

For example, at one point I was struggling with a plan to do a very enjoyable thirty-minute online stretch routine every Sunday morning when I woke up. I knew this habit was one I wanted to adopt, since it was one where I could wake up whenever I wanted and do something that made my body feel good during and after. But despite this, I hadn't been able to keep it up. I knew there wasn't anything deeper to it than just forgetting about it as an action. So, I decided to transfer some speed bumps from Sunday morning to Saturday to create a plan of less resistance. I put an alarm on my phone that reminded me to do two things on Saturday in preparation for Sunday:

1. Charge my iPad and load up the guided stretching video

2. Put my yoga mat somewhere visible ready for the morning

Then, when I woke up on Sunday, I had to walk over a giant yellow mat to get from bed to coffee in the morning, which I absolutely noticed and remembered why it was there.

Sweet spots

When helping clients to reintroduce foods that they initially choose to cut out because they feel out of control around them, I encourage them to adopt what I call 'sweet spot' thinking. It's aligned with previous themes around illogical reasoning when it comes to eating behaviours.

I learned, while identifying my ideal way of eating, that the foods I didn't seem to think I could eat in small amounts weren't actually most enjoyable to me the large amounts I thought I wanted to consume them in. I was going by the logic that if the first slice of cake is delicious and the second is also delicious, then the fifth must still be delicious. When in fact, after the first couple of slices, the rewards started diminishing in terms of how much I was enjoying the experience. Not only because of side effects like bloating or feeling hyper, but because the fifteenth bite is completely different to the first bite. This realisation helped me identify the distinction between using and abusing foods that I haven't previously been able to consume in reasonable amounts.

If you think you could do with developing more 'sweet spot' thinking, cast your mind back to the last moment you had during a meal when you thought, 'I am truly enjoying this eating experience. This food is genuinely delicious.' Then consider:

How much had you eaten?

At what stage of the meal was it that you were you most enjoying your food?

Then, try to be more mindful of this concept as you go about your daily life making choices about when to stop eating.

Post-binge reactivation plan

If like me, you've been known to suffer with seriously uncomfortable post-binge withdrawals, I have an extra tip I'd like to share with you. For me and many of my clients, the first couple of days into a healthier diet after a stretch of heavily bingeing on unhealthy food is incredibly difficult physically, and can involve anything from pounding headaches and acid reflux to skin outbreaks and anxiety.

If you find yourself in a situation where, for whatever reason, you feel that physical withdrawals are holding you back from pushing through the first few days of a new eating plan and coming out the other side, then I recommend creating a little pre-activation plan that involves committing to just three days of general physical preparation before focusing on weight management.

For me, this involves steadily decreasing my intake of the foods I want to cut out while creating comfortable conditions to ride out my withdrawals in. For example, I will decide that for three days I will only snack on unlimited amounts on fruit that I enjoy, make sure I drink three litres of water and, when it comes to meals, eat things that I know won't leave me craving more soon after. I won't focus on losing weight yet, just on feeling less unwell and less full of physical urges for starchy foods or those that are high in sugar. Then, when it gets to re-activation day, things don't seem nearly as difficult. Any further cravings and urges become considerably more tolerable because I am no longer swimming against the very strong current of physical withdrawal.

Now you know what you need to know about the lapsing process, I'd like to help you create a couple of extra tools that will help further minimise the likelihood of unwanted lapses.

Written Exercise: Early Warning Signs

First, think about subtle ways in which you might start neglecting your commitment to your plan and giving your goals less importance. These are things to be on alert for going forward. Sometimes one or two at a time can be fine but when a few are allowed to worsen gradually and continue to add up however subtly for too long, plans can start derailing without us noticing.

1. _____

2. _____

3. _____

4. _____

5. _____

6. _____

E.g. Not completing my AM check-in, justifying why a blip should drag on, not making sure I review my plan regularly, isolating and not connecting with friends and family who make me feel positive

Map: Emergency Plan

First, write 'Emergency Plan' in the middle of a blank page and draw a circle around it. Now think of someone who you'd happily take advice from because you know they have your best interests at heart. Someone who cares deeply about your happiness and really wants to help you achieve your goals. They know your history well and they know exactly what you need to hear to stay on track using the tools and exercises you've picked up. Imagine you have bumped into this person either during or en route to an unwanted lapse. You tell them what's going on, and the combination of guidance, advice and reminders they give you convinces you to get back on track immediately. On your map, write down what they said, drawing a circle around each response as you go.

When you're finished, what you have in front of you is a snapshot of bespoke take-aways from this process that you can glance at all at once. It will provide you with the bounce-back guidance that gives you the greatest chance of getting back on track with a challenging eating plan ASAP.

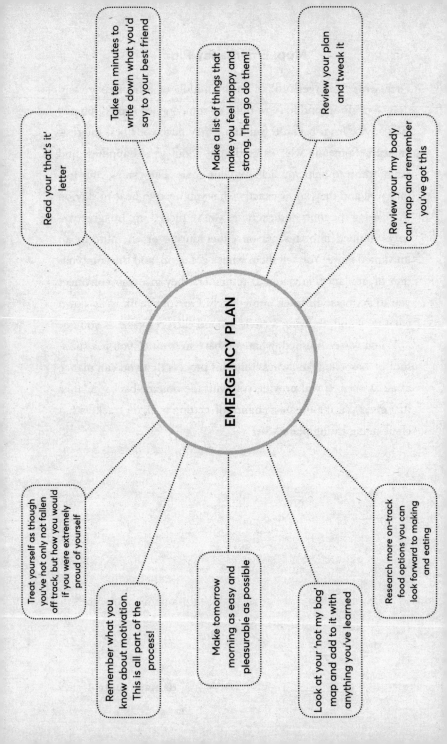

EMERGENCY PLAN

Read your 'that's it' letter

Take ten minutes to write down what you'd say to your best friend

Make a list of things that make you feel happy and strong. Then go do them!

Review your plan and tweak it

Review your 'my body can' map and remember you've got this

Research more on-track food options you can look forward to making and eating

Look at your 'not my bag' map and add to it with anything you've learned

Make tomorrow morning as easy and pleasurable as possible

Remember what you know about motivation. This is all part of the process!

Treat yourself as though you've not only not fallen off track, but how you would if you were extremely proud of yourself

kind control

People often ask me how I can be so confident that I won't go back to my old ways. The simple truth is, I've made it unappealing for myself to do so, because:

- I've got a default 'healthy way of eating' I'm happy with that I now generally stick to without much thought. Any spontaneous decisions to deviate from it are conscious and I never regret them

- Since my body has always been prone to gaining weight quickly, I now accept that I will fluctuate in size throughout my life, and that's OK. Recently I went to Italy for ten days and joyfully ate in a way that would quite frankly make anyone gain weight. But I didn't beat myself up about this for a second. Not just because I recognised an opportunity to truly enjoy eating for the glorious experience that it is, or because I don't beat myself up about anything anymore. Mainly because I knew that I had a bespoke, effective weight-management plan waiting for me when I got home

- My response to even a tiny bit of weight gain is the opposite of what it was before. Now, I ramp up my self-care and ensure that I wear clothes that make me feel great and speak to myself in my most encouraging of voices. Before I know it I'm back at the weight I'm happy with

- When my body craves a behaviour pattern my mind knows I want to break in any area of my life, I observe it like a child who can't be blamed for wanting what it wants but whose demands simply won't be obeyed. I acknowledge it with compassion and understanding without feeling at the mercy of it. This has helped me feel incredibly capable of impulse control across a range of life areas

- I like how my body looks and feels, and that makes me feel strong and happy as a new baseline every day. I'm so aware of the habits that move me away from feeling like this that it's become a no-brainer not to engage in them

- If I wake up feeling bloated, I see it as just that. It's not a signal that I may as well keep eating bloating and fattening foods because I don't like how I look

- I place importance on how I see myself behaving when no one else is watching. If I don't feel happy with any behaviour I engage in, that's enough to make me want to change it. I don't need anyone else to witness my actions for me to want to change them

- I've done so many 'Gig's Up'-style maps that there are no more excuses or variations on excuses left to entertain, and now any new ones don't really stand a chance against my internal bullshit detector

- Whether it's a decision about what I'll eat or how I respond to an email that has angered me, I've taught myself through weight management to automatically project into the future and ask how I'll wish I behaved tomorrow and next week

- I am on a mission in every aspect of my life to reduce the time it takes to forgive myself for anything I didn't mean to do or later wish I hadn't done

- When I'm not sure whether an act towards my body is a kind one, I automatically consider what choice I'd want my mum to make for herself in that moment

- I have entirely new automatic self-care habits that were adopted not to remedy something, but purely to increase my enjoyment and wellbeing. They are absolutely a part of my daily routine and play an enormous part in me feeling happy with the day-to-day decisions I make across all areas of my life, including food. When I'm not behaving kindly towards myself in any way, I notice immediately

- I catch the moments when my first impulse to soothe or comfort myself is to eat food as opposed to trying a different coping strategy. If someone upsets me and I catch myself wanting to reach for something sugary, I can distinguish this from hunger. It's become such an obvious distinction now that I hear myself internally saying things like, 'I bet if you don't get the response you want to that text you'll immediately think you're hungry even though you just ate lunch.' It's become like an observation game of my thoughts and feelings, and I'm fully aware that they don't have to dictate my actions

- I genuinely enjoy keeping up my new kinder eating habits. These days, the fact they contribute to weight management is a bonus. I like striving every day to build a kinder, more positive internal and external world for myself, especially when it's challenging. One where acts and thoughts of unkindness are not welcome and stick out like a sore thumb. I'm finding it easier than I could ever have imagined to maintain my weight, because it makes me feel good to do so. After all, that's all The Last Diet was really ever about: finally learning to feel good in and about myself so I could make decisions on the spot about any part of my life that are in my best interests.

Now it's your turn.